PSYCHIATRISTS ON PSYCHIATRY

PSYCHIATRISTS ON PSYCHIATRY

Edited by
MICHAEL SHEPHERD
Professor of Epidemiological Psychiatry,
Institute of Psychiatry, University of London

CAMBRIDGE UNIVERSITY PRESS
Cambridge
London New York New Rochelle
Melbourne Sydney

CAMBRIDGE UNIVERSITY PRESS
Cambridge, New York, Melbourne, Madrid, Cape Town, Singapore, São Paulo, Delhi

Cambridge University Press
The Edinburgh Building, Cambridge CB2 8RU, UK

Published in the United States of America by Cambridge University Press, New York

www.cambridge.org
Information on this title: www.cambridge.org/9780521288637

First published 1982
Re-issued in this digitally printed version 2009

A catalogue record for this publication is available from the British Library

Library of Congress Catalogue Card Number: 81-21750

ISBN 978-0-521-24480-0 hardback
ISBN 978-0-521-28863-7 paperback

CONTENTS

CONTRIBUTORS

Prof. M. Bleuler, Bahnhofstrasse 49, Zollikon, Zurich, Switzerland CH–8702

Dr A. W. Clare, Institute of Psychiatry, De Crespigny Park, London SE5 8AF, England

Prof. R. R. Grinker Sr, Institute for Psychosomatic and Psychiatric Research and Training, Michael Reese Hospital and Medical Center, 29th Street and Ellis Avenue, Chicago, Illinois 60616, USA

Dr H. Häfner, Zentralinstitut für Seelische Gesundheit Mannheim, 6800 Mannheim 1, 15 Postfach 5970, Germany

Dr A. Jablensky, Division of Mental Health, World Health Organisation, 1211 Geneva 27, Switzerland

Prof. S. S. Kety, The Mailman Research Center, The McLean Hospital, 115 Mill Street, Belmont, Mass. 02178, USA

Dr T. A. Lambo, World Health Organisation, 1211 Geneva 27, Switzerland

Prof. P. Pichot, Centre Hospitalier Saint Anne, 100 Rue de la Santé, 75671, Paris, Cedex 14, France

Prof. J. Romano, School of Medicine and Psychiatry and Strong Memorial Hospital, University of Rochester, 300 Crittenden Boulevard, Rochester, New York 14642, USA

Prof. E. Strömgren, University of Aarhus Psychiatric Hospital, DK–8230 Risskov, Denmark

Prof. H. Strotzka, Institut für Tiefenpsychologie und Psychotherapie der Universität Wien, A–1090 Wien, Lazarettgasse 14, Austria

Dr D. C. Watt, St John's Hospital, Stone, Aylesbury, Buckinghamshire, England

INTRODUCTION

'The future of psychiatry in science and society' was the title of a recent lecture delivered by an eminent British neurophysiologist[1]. While acknowledging his lay status, he justified his choice of topic by claiming that '... psychiatry is public property. It is, like no other area of medicine, thought about, agonised over, discussed and criticised, by people who have no direct contact with it as a medical discipline either as practitioners or sufferers.' A persuasive explanation of this observation, which has been made often enough elsewhere, has been provided by a French commentator: 'Placée à l'intersection des besoins clinico-thérapeutiques, des sciences humaines et de la demande sociale, la psychiatrié est devenue l'objet privilegié de grands débats ou s'incarnent certaines des interrogations les plus aiguës liées aux évolutions et à la crise culturelle de notre temps'[2]. It is not surprising, therefore, that in recent years the subject-matter of psychiatry has become fair game not only for neurobiologists but also for a host of other groups and factions in the psychological and social sciences, the mass media, the arts, politics, philosophy, religion, fringe medicine and cults of all description, not least the anti-psychiatry movement.

Yet all too often these cacophonous, and mostly ill-informed, discussions have tended to minimise or ignore the fact that psychiatry, like all other medical disciplines, is organised around what Talcott Parsons called 'the application of scientific knowledge by technically competent, trained personnel'. The great majority of its medically trained workers are hard-working physicians, more concerned with narrow professional preoccupations than with the broader implications of their activities. In consequence, the voice of the central figure in modern psychiatry, the practising psychiatrist, is rarely heard by the public at large. It seemed, therefore, that a collective expression of their points of view was overdue: hence, this collection of essays.

A word about the structure and composition of the volume is in order. While a compilation of this size cannot, of course, claim to be comprehensive, the 12 participants – who include some of the most outstanding and

[1] Blakemore, C. (1981). The future of psychiatry in science and society. *Psychological Medicine*, 11, 27–38.
[2] Introduction to *Domaines de la Psychiatrié* (1980). Paris: Privat.

best-known contemporary psychiatrists – were chosen to sample variations in age, nationality, background, experience and theoretical standpoint in an attempt to provide a reasonably representative cross-section of current opinion. Other collections of essays on or by prominent psychiatrists have tended to concentrate on biographical or autobiographical accounts in a more or less unstructured manner. Here, each author was invited to follow the same format in his contribution, consisting of a brief personal sketch and an outline of professional experience and influences, followed by an assessment of the current status of the discipline and its future prospects. On the basis of this material, three points were selected for further comment in the form of question and answer.

The result is revealing and instructive. More than 100 years after the publication of Griesinger's *Mental Pathology*, which Ludwig Binswanger justly termed the 'Magna Carta' of psychiatry, it is evident that opinion is unanimous on several major aspects of its development: the need to preserve the connection with general medicine, the importance of fostering research, a disillusionment with psychoanalysis and the resistance to the anti-psychiatric trends of recent years. Widely differing notions, however, are entertained on other central issues, including the relevance of psychiatry to social policy, the desirable directions of its future evolution and the role of the biological sciences in the causation of mental disease.

While these differences may be attributed as much to emphasis and perspective as to substance and ideology, they also reflect in some measure the vantage-point of the observer. It is not always recalled that psychiatry is practised in three quite different settings: the mental hospital, the general hospital and the various community services. A glance at the contributions of Professor Bleuler, Professor Strömgren and Dr Watt, all of whom have worked in the mental hospital milieu for most of their professional lives, indicates an overriding awareness of the problems of institutional care and of that large segment of the psychiatric population which continues to need it. By contrast, Professor Häfner, Professor Strotzka, Dr Jablensky, Dr Lambo and Dr Clare are all, in their different ways, chiefly orientated towards the social and community facets of psychiatry. Yet again, the strong links with neurology and general medicine forged by Professors Grinker and Romano understandably render them more concerned with those features of psychiatry which are prominent in a more medical context, while the outlook of Professors Kety and Pichot represents the approach of the increasing number of psychobiological scientists who are concerning themselves with the problems of mental disease.

Introduction

From the rich variety of the contributors' views and experience the content of psychiatry emerges as a complex omnium gatherum. Their essays as a group indicate the process of fragmentation that underlies the confusing and often self-contradictory assessments of the subject by its own practitioners, reflecting the high degree of specialisation demanded of a growing body of knowledge that draws heavily on many other disciplines. Also, they suggest that the time may be ripe for a serious attempt from within the profession to integrate the loose federation of facts, theories and concepts that have developed so profusely in the last four decades. In this way the profession should be able to take stock of achievements, identify areas requiring further work and respond more convincingly to the questions, speculations and fantasies of the interested lay public. Psychiatry may well be too important a topic to leave to the psychiatrists, but there is no reason for them to refrain from a more concerted effort designed to map the direction of their own work and to become more aware of its implications. If this book does no more than help to provide guidelines, it will have served a useful purpose.

MICHAEL SHEPHERD

Institute of Psychiatry,
London, 1981

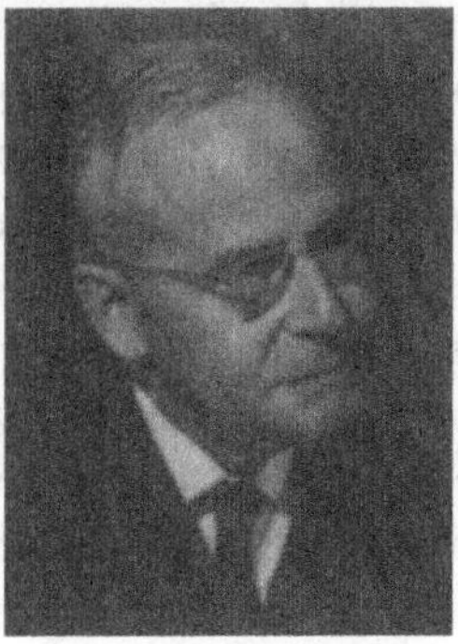

1 · MANFRED BLEULER

Personal background and professional experience

All my father's ancestors lived in Zollikon near Zurich. Until the beginning of this century Zollikon was a small country village with a farming population. Following the Age of Enlightenment in the eighteenth century the inhabitants experienced a growing interest in intellectual matters and libraries were collected in farmhouses. The intellectual needs of the population were, however, frustrated until my grandfather's time, as access to higher education was a privilege restricted to the citizens of Zurich. The rural population felt that the clergymen, physicians, judges and public functionaries assigned to work in the country were not up to their duties. The hope grew that the farmers' own sons would do better. Nevertheless, it took a long time after the inauguration of the University of Zurich in 1833, open as it was to the whole population, for intellectuals from the country to be acknowledged as the equals of the aristocratic citizens.

The tension became particularly great in the field of psychiatry. The first University Professors of Psychiatry, who were also the first Directors of the University Clinic of Burghölzli near Zollikon (inaugurated in 1870), were highly qualified psychiatrists, such as Von Gudden and Hitzig. As Zurich at that time had no academic tradition, professors from Germany were appointed to chairs of psychiatry. The rural population in the vicinity of the Clinic felt that these men were too distant from the patients and too much interested in laboratory work. They also felt markedly resentful of the professors' use of German rather than the patients' mother tongue, the Zurich dialect. The people believed that a psychiatrist who spoke the patients' mother tongue would understand the patients' worries, ailments and hopes better than a foreign scientist. It was generally expected that one of their own sons would spend all his time near his patients, speak with them and become their real doctor.

This idealistic background provided the stimulus for my father (born in 1857) to study medicine and to become a psychiatrist in the Zurich psychiatric Clinic. His main contribution to psychiatry accorded well with such a mission: he studied the content, the meaning of his patients' utterances and their psychodynamic life, rather than a static psychopathology. Only late in life did I realise how much a calling, rooted in the minds of my ancestors' community, has also influenced the course of my own development.

My mother was the daughter of an intellectual citizen of Zurich. Her father died when she was young and she found her favourite home during vacations in the farmhouse of her mother's parents. She was the first Zurich girl to study languages and history, and she became a teacher at the girls' college.

From 1879 to 1898 August Forel, a very passionate fighter for social reforms and against alcoholism, was Professor of Psychiatry in Zurich. All his pupils, including my father (who had been his resident physician in 1885), were on his side and many citizens joined his group. My parents met during this teamwork. They were married in 1901 and enjoyed a happy marriage until my father's death in 1939.

I was born in 1903 in my parents' apartment in the Zurich psychiatric Clinic, where I spent my entire childhood and adolescence in close contact with patients. My siblings and I were taught to participate in many of the patients' activities: for instance, I used to engage in theatricals with them.

I went to school in Zurich and passed the Federal entrance examination for the University of Zurich. I spent the first year of my medical studies in Geneva, in order to become acquainted with the French way of life. My further medical studies were mainly carried out at the University of Zurich. I obtained my medical degree in 1927 and my doctorate of medicine in 1929.

In my adolescence my main interests lay in biology and mathematics. At the age of 15 I worked out a childish 'research project' on a possible correlation between the frequency of different species of butterflies and the frequency of the plants feeding their caterpillars in a region bounded by a lake and high rocks. I worked out clumsy correlation coefficients and 'discovered' that there was no such association. During my time at college a small group of boys discussed biological problems. At that time Mendelism had been rediscovered in biology and was introduced into psychiatry. An entomologist at our University named Standfuss introduced me to cross-breed butterflies; he was successful in distinguishing between hereditary and environmental influences on the colours and designs of the butterfly-wings. I then studied the transmission of albinism and colours in cross-breeding rabbits and we discussed the results. We also made experiments on the placebo effect of drugs.

My summarized biography after graduation as a physician is as follows. In 1928 I was intern and from 1930 to 1932 First Assistant at the Kantonsspital Liestal, a 120-bed country hospital catering mostly for surgical and obstetrical patients. Between my two periods of duty there I was in America for 18 months working at the Boston Psychopathic Hospital, at the neurological service of the Boston City Hospital and at the Bloomingdale Hospital in White Plains, New York. In 1932, while mountain climbing, I broke my cervical spine and suffered a spinal haemorrhage with paraplegia. During convalescence I worked at the children's service of the Burghölzli Clinic. As the spasticity of my left side persisted I had to give up surgery and became part-time Oberarzt at the Psychiatric Clinic at St Pirminsberg, in the mountains. There I also did part-time general practice in the Alpine valley above the Clinic (1933–8).

Between 1938 and 1942 I was Chief Physician at the Psychiatric University Clinic in Basle and became a lecturer in psychiatry at the University. From the beginning of World War II, however, I was mostly on military service as a battalion surgeon in the army. From 1942 to 1969 I was Professor of Psychiatry at the University of Zurich and Director of the Psychiatric University Clinic of Burghölzli, a 550-bed hospital, catering chiefly for severe psychotics, but with an outpatient department, a family care organisation and a children's service. In 1969 I retired from my position and have been treating private patients and writing since.

I married Monica Bisaz in 1946. She had been a nurse and came from the Engadine, a mountain valley with its own culture and language, which became very dear to me. She has helped me in all my work, becoming a friend of my patients and participating in my research work. We have one daughter, who has studied agriculture and is eager to improve the farmers' living conditions in the Alps.

When I was a small child, C. G. Jung and his family lived in the apartment above ours in Burghölzli and his children were my playmates.

I noticed early the interest displayed by Jung and my father in our behaviour. This experience had some indirect influence on my later psychological interests. Many years later I realised that Jung and my father had tested the early teachings of Freud on us and had mentioned some of these observations in their papers.

It is self-evident that my attitude to psychiatry was influenced by my father. When writing this account I realise that he never lectured on psychiatry to me, nor did his main influence come from his books. What impressed me most was watching his contacts with patients. In his talks with them, he and his patients were entirely concentrated on each other and they seemed to me to form a close and friendly community.

During college days Hermann Rorschach worked in a hospital near Zurich and frequently came to discuss his early work with my father. They tested the members of our family and I had to test my school-fellows. I always listened carefully to their discussions. I have never lost my interest in projection tests, but I do not accept the illusion that they can reduce the characteristics of a man to a formula. Nonetheless, they have helped me to discover hidden intellectual and imaginative capacities in patients who had seemed to be superficial and uninteresting. I devoted my thesis to the study of similarities of the Rorschach test results in siblings and of whether these depended on environmental or hereditary influences. Later I and my brother, a farmer in Morocco, studied illiterate Moroccans by means of the test.

While working in general hospitals I never lost interest in the patients' personalities and living conditions. My surgical chief, Arnold Berger, was a master at taking into account the personalities of his patients.

I became familiar with Adolf Meyer's common sense psychiatry on the occasion of his visits to my father. I also watched the practical side of Meyer's teaching in America, where I enjoyed the enthusiasm for research and the absence of the over-critical attitude I had met too frequently in Europe. The open-hearted way I was accepted among the interns and residents in American hospitals made me happy and led to lifelong friendships. I learned much from my psychiatric and neurological chiefs, Macfie C. Campbell, Stanley Cobb and Mortimer Raynor. As an intern of Stanley Cobb I had to examine patients under the care of Harvey Cushing. His great interest in the psychopathology of his patients with basophil adenomata of the pituitary stimulated my own interest in endocrinological psychiatry. In endocrinology lies a synthesis of somatic and psychological medicine that has always intrigued me and I wished to survey the whole field.

Personal background and professional experience

During my 27½ years as a professor and Clinic Director in Zurich I devoted all my time to the patients, to the students and to research. The possibilities of research were limited by my routine duties and were restricted to periods of leave from the hospital. One most productive leave was spent at Oskar Diethelm's clinic at New York Hospital, others amid the lovely scenery of Smaland in Sweden. Within the hospital, patients, staff and I myself enjoyed a good life together and the students seemed to be interested in my eight carefully prepared lectures a week. The concentration on the hospital, on teaching and on some research in my free time demanded great sacrifices, forcing me to neglect my relations with the government and the public, and to neglect fund-raising and collaboration with other faculty members, the University and psychiatric societies. Dismayed at the thought of all I have neglected I have only one excuse: it was impossible to do everything and concentration on my main task was my first duty.

There were two exceptions to this precept. First, I felt it my duty to our army to study and to teach military psychology. And, secondly, I presided over the second World Congress of Psychiatry in 1957 at Zurich, which I organised with Werner Stoll as Secretary.

My main research concerns the long-term course of schizophrenic psychoses, the whole life history of schizophrenics and the factors acting upon them including the influence of therapy, family members, constitution and physical health. I started these studies in 1929 in Boston and am still involved with them. Two of the many conclusions were important for me: the general prognosis is better than was previously believed, and even the chronic patients do not deteriorate as a rule. Indeed, from the fifth year of the psychosis they tend to improve. Our therapy had often been considered to be symptomatic and many believe that it will be replaced by a 'real', causal therapy as soon as the nature of the psychosis is discovered. I am now convinced that we already know much in regard to its nature. Our knowledge makes it possible for us to consider our therapy as adequate in relation to the genesis of the psychosis, as causal and highly important and meriting further development and application with a sense of conviction: we should incorporate the patient in active communities, secure the possibilities of using his capacities and calm him if the psychosis is too painful for him or if a state of excitation becomes dangerous.

Confronted with an ever-increasing amount of knowledge, the growing number of publications and the increasing sub-division of psychiatry into sub-specialities, I have tried in my teaching and in successive reviews of my father's textbook to keep in mind the basic facts of psychology and psychiatry and to demonstrate that the essentials can be clearly summarised.

Since retiring from the hospital I have continued to see patients at my home. Most of my long-planned books have been published recently: the English translation of the monograph on schizophrenic psychoses, a summary of endocrinological psychiatry, a history of the research carried out at Burghölzli and the fourteenth edition of my father's textbook. My wife and I enjoy the natural environment and are much engaged in the fight for the protection of nature and natural resources.

Current status of psychiatry

Since World War II the status of psychiatry has been contested. Every psychiatrist and large sections of the population are aware of this trend which the mass media publicise blatantly.

An important reason for the defamation of psychiatry was the miserable state of hospital conditions: too many psychiatric hospitals in too many countries were or still are understaffed, overcrowded, poorly planned and financially impoverished. While two centuries ago most hospitals were forms of poor-houses, hospitals for somatic illness have long been adapted to reach higher medical standards and to create modern living conditions. The psychiatric hospitals have, by contrast, lagged far behind and are still backward in many places. The psychiatrists' struggle for better hospitals has too often proved unsuccessful, and for too long the public and governmental idea prevailed that psychiatric hospitals were only for the segregation of the 'insane' and should cost as little as possible. The old, unfavourable image of psychiatric hospitals is still to be found, even where the institutions have been modernised.

We are now witnessing a turning of the tide, but if we adapt life in 'mental health centres' to the life of an open welfare society (an ambitious undertaking!) we are in danger of neglecting the needs of the most difficult and most helpless patients. It is easy enough to create a pleasant climate in a psychiatric centre if we exclude from admission the untidiest, the most aggressive and the most chronic patients. And it is not difficult to diminish the number of hospital inmates if one does not care for the discharged chronic patients and fails to secure their welfare. There is still a frightening gap between the pleasant image of a paradisial mental health centre, from which every patient is quickly discharged, and the cruel reality of the population of chronic patients for whom we have to care, many of them helpless, noisy, untidy or aggressive. We are in need of progress in the synthesis of care for the chronic *and* the acute, the most difficult *and* the most tractable patients. It is a noble mission to include in our duties the care of patients suffering from such conditions as senile dementia, epileptic deterioration or high-grade mental deficiency.

Authority is vanishing in our society today. It is no longer self-evident that the physician assumes the responsibility for a patient who cannot assess his own needs, who cannot care for himself and risks starvation or death without help. Must we hospitalise him, if necessary, feed him, treat him – even if the patient cannot give his consent? If the physician does so, he risks being accused of infringing the patient's human rights; if he does not, he becomes guilty of neglecting his patient. We are in need of clearer definitions of the psychiatrist's rights and duties in helping patients who are unable to judge reality or exercise realistic volition.

Confronted with the huge number of new psychiatric research results and publications, with the increasingly complex, sophisticated languages of many psychiatric fields, a general survey of psychiatry became difficult. We are starting to realise, however, that psychiatry does not consist essentially of an amassment of overspecialised knowledge and hypotheses: its basic facts are astonishingly clear and simple. What is going on in psychotherapy, for instance, is of the same nature as what is going on in any relationship with other people. It is an urgent task of present-day psychiatry to disclose the basic facts of human life, to survey and summarise detailed knowledge, and again to find a clear and simple language with which to express ourselves.

Psychiatric help is needed everywhere, but every kind of psychiatric method is not adequate for every population. There is a growing danger of our imposing our Western psychiatry on people of other civilisations. Not all psychiatric therapies are universally effective in the way, for example, that anti-thyroid drugs are used for the psychosis associated with thyrotoxicosis, or nicotinic acid for the psychosis of pellagra. Many other therapies have to be adapted to local traditions, local customs, local faiths and local social structures: these include the therapies in psychiatric hospitals and psychiatric centres, group therapy, social therapy and even personal psychotherapy. As psychiatrists we should be pioneers in respecting tradition and the way of life of alien peoples and social groups.

Future prospects of psychiatry

The future of psychiatry depends on the future of medicine and, I dare to add, the future of medicine on the future of psychiatry. Both are threatened today.

At all times and in all cultures with which we are familiar 'our doctor' is the man or the woman on whom we can rely in peeriods of physical and mental distress. He is the man we can call to our bedside in states of torment and desperation. We know he will come. We realise that he cannot cure every disease, but we know that he helps in the best way possible. To know that he is near, to feel that his whole attention, mind and heart are engaged to provide help, constitutes in itself a great source of solace for the sick, even if physical measures are of no assistance.

Today there are many other characteristics of a physician which render him indispensable: to him, and only to him, can we demonstrate our ailments and reveal our bodily and moral nakedness. He will accept our misery naturally, without exhibiting blame, derision or disgust. And even more: his knowledge of our most intimate concerns does not involve us in any long-lasting dependence. We are free to terminate contact with our doctor whenever we no longer need him. The doctor is bound by professional secrecy. We are sure that he has successfully gone through a long and hard professional training.

The traditional relationship between the patient and the doctor is unique in its way, close and clearly delimited. Medicine is no longer medicine if the traditional concept of a doctor is lost. Unfortunately, it is now in danger of disappearing. The personal physician's beneficial influence radiates from him personally. Today more and more specialists are needed for more and more diseases. The individual doctor's influence vanishes if several specialists care for one patient. Team-work among specialists should be better organised than is now usual: only one of them should take over the task of the patient's personal doctor and the others should be consultants, providing background advice. More and more physicians are increasingly fascinated by impersonal medical interests, by technical problems, by laboratory findings or by research. The patient, however, becomes lonely and risks losing the beneficial influence emanating from his own physician. Who replaces him? Frequently, no one at all. Nurses are also becoming more and more specialised and more and more distant from the patient. All too often it is in consequence the untrained nurse or the maid who becomes the hospital patient's confidante.

The danger hanging over medicine has been well illustrated by the petition of two surgeons, experts in a sub-specialty, who wanted the hospital to engage a psychologist to undertake the task of speaking to the patients. If physicians need psychologists to speak to their patients, if they are technicians, biologists, researchers or teachers rather than doctors close to the patient, then the traditional figure of the doctor is vanishing, and with it the doctor's important psychological influence on the patient. At the same time medicine, which has been a noble field of human activity (with an undisputedly didactic role), will be split into different components. Psychologists, technicians, biologists, social workers and many other professionals will increasingly take over the traditional tasks of the physician.

If the figure of the personal doctor is no longer rooted in the deepest feelings of his patients, the psychiatrist can be replaced by trained psychologists, social workers and several other professionals who will have to collaborate with him. By virtue of his status as a physician, however, the psychiatrist enjoys a particular opportunity to act as a psychotherapist. His patient knows, of course, that he does not practise surgery, obstetrics or other somatic specialities, but he also knows that he has had a training in general medicine. He has therefore an understanding of many medical problems and he is better able to make a synthesis of his patients' somatic and psychological personality than anyone else. It is hard to imagine how the psychiatrist as a doctor could be replaced. If the psychiatrist is no longer a physician, the concept of psychiatry loses its meaning. Psychiatry can subsist only if medicine survives.

Unfortunately, it seems probable that the dissolution of psychiatry may precede the dissolution of medicine and medical representation. For different reasons psychiatry is more exposed by present-day developments than somatic medicine: psychotherapy, the most important form of psychiatric therapy, was developed by physicians but is claimed now to be the province of non-medical psychologists, social workers and other professionals. Even more dangerous for the future of psychiatry, however, is the way in which psychiatrists themselves are turning from their patients. One of the deplorable signs of this trend is the tendency to explore the patient's personality by questionnaires and test-batteries instead of learning to know him by talking to and being with him. The contemporary psychiatrist is tempted to spend much time on administrative duties, on public relations or on laboratory research, lecturing and writing. It is, of course, necessary for the well-being of the discipline that many psychiatrists are also teachers and research-workers, but if the majority of them find teaching and research more important than the provision of personal help for their patients, then psychiatrists will leave their rightful place close to their patients and the decline of their subject will follow.

And what would medicine be without psychiatry? It would hardly survive. Physicians would be forced to seek advice from non-medical professionals who would move closer to the patients and become their confidantes. The physician would be the traditional doctor no longer, and what could medicine be without a doctor as the patient's confidante?

It is possible that medicine, the concept of the traditional doctor and psychiatry as a medical discipline will disappear in future societies. It is impossible, however, to imagine how medicine and the traditional doctor could be replaced without harm to mankind. If we wish to preserve medicine and psychiatry for future generations it is an urgent task for all physicians, and for psychiatrists in particular, to be personally involved with the sick and to devote most of their endeavours to remaining close to the patient himself.

Questions and answers

1. You say of schizophrenia: 'I am now convinced that we already know much in regard to its nature.' Would you elaborate on your views concerning aetiology?

(a) Since the beginning of this century many new research findings in general physiology and in brain physiology have led to speculation concerning their possible significance in the understanding of the aetiology of schizophrenia. Up to now, however, it has not been possible to establish any somatic substrate for schizophrenia. I have, of course, studied the dopamine and endorphin hypotheses but their proponents have not yet demonstrated that any change in the metabolism of dopamine or the endorphins constitutes an essential basis for the schizophrenic psychoses.

Confronted with these negative findings many research workers, while retaining a belief in the somatic basis of the schizophrenic psychoses, have questioned whether their methods are yet sufficiently refined to detect its nature. This viewpoint is justifiable. I think, however, that we should also consider the alternative: that it has not been discovered because it does not exist! In medicine we must look for a preliminary understanding of an illness on the grounds of what we know, rather than rely on speculations. We must accept, therefore, the possibility that the development of schizophrenia takes place in the human psychic life, in spheres and dimensions whose somatic background we are unable to perceive, in the same spheres and dimensions where the neurotic and the healthy personality develop as a result of the interwoven influences of inherited disposition and life experience. This notion does not mean that schizophrenia is a neurosis: it is very different from neurosis in its psychopathological and social aspects but not, perhaps, in respect of the elusive nature of a somatic background.

(**b**) Though it is certain that hereditary disposition plays a role in aetiology, neither a Mendelian transmission of a schizophrenic gene nor an hereditary metabolic error has ever been demonstrated. A reasonable assumption is that the hereditary background for schizophrenia is a dysharmony of hereditary disposition for the development of the personality, of the ego. This realistic hypothesis permits us to hope that we may find a causal therapy for schizophrenia even if we fail to find a metabolic error.

(**c**) It is certain that many life experiences, particularly those connected with members of the patient's family, play a role in the development of schizophrenia.

(**d**) If we study schizophrenic patients very carefully we observe the importance of interaction between the difficult personality and stressful life experience. The psychosis develops when the conflicts between the patient's own drives, and between his drives and his social environment, become overwhelming: from this moment on he denies realistic experience and logical thinking to inhabit an autistic world of phantasy which is better adapted to his contradictory self than is reality. What we discover in the course of extended psychotherapy with a schizophrenic might be considered today as the essential pointer to the aetiology of schizophrenia. Such a notion, however, is not the clue to the understanding of every problem; it hardly explains, for instance, the phasic or schizo-affective psychoses.

(**e**) The course of the psychosis is clearly different from the course of cerebral diseases. It corresponds to the aforementioned model.

(**f**) What is effective in the treatment of schizophrenics is also effective in the development of the healthy individual: clear and steady personal relations, activity in accord with one's talents, interests and strength, confrontation with new responsibilities or even with dangers and the appropriate rhythm between activity and relaxation. The same influences which develop the healthy ego are the main therapy for the split ego. This therapeutic experience argues in favour of the assumption that schizophrenia develops in the same spheres as the normal human personality.

2. In the opinion of some authorities the role which you attribute to the psychiatrist in the latter part of your chapter belongs rightly to the general practitioner. How do you view this contention?

I do believe that the everyday work of a psychiatrist and of a general practitioner overlap. They will overlap more in the future, as minor surgery and obstetrics pass increasingly from the general practitioner to specialists. The general practitioner must be more and more a psychotherapist in the sense that I have mentioned. The psychiatrist, however, must be an expert not only in psychotherapy, but also in somatic medicine: he must, for example, understand the physical side-effects of psychotropic drugs, know when an ailment might be an expression of an emotion and when somatic diagnostic measures are indicated, and appreciate the consequences of cerebral and endocrine diseases on the emotions. In this sense he must be as much of a physician as the general practitioner and in one sense even more so, because his status as a doctor is a good background for his psychotherapy. Yet, although their responsibilities overlap, the main fields of activities undertaken by the psychiatrist and the general practitioner will be different: the general practitioner will inevitably have more to do with somatic medicine, while the psychiatrist will be more interested in long-term psychotherapy, social psychiatry and some particular psychotherapeutic techniques. Many patients will decide themselves whether to consult the psychiatrist or the general practitioner.

3. How do you reconcile the claims made by biological scientists with your opinion of psychiatry's basic facts?

I am aware, of course, of the rich variety of research findings in modern biology and brain physiology, anatomy and chemistry. I admire the complicated and difficult techniques used by modern biologists. I think, however, that the significance of all this knowledge for psychology and psychiatry can be summarised and expressed in a few clear and impressive theses; we should neglect sophisticated, uncertain speculations and keep to the main facts and to well-elaborated theories. Such a summary should point out principally the probable relationships between the neurotransmitters at the neural synapses and activation, sedation and mood changes; the interaction between nervous, endocrinological and emotional functions; the functions of cerebral systems which regulate primitive drives such as hunger, thirst, breeding instincts and sexuality; and the significance of the oxygen supply to the brain. It should bring together a few of the theories on memory; and it should mention what we know and do not know with regard to the localisation of elementary psychological functions.

Select bibliography

Bleuler, M. (1928). Der Rorschach'sche Formdeutversuch bei Geschwistern. *Z. Neurol.*, **118**, 366–98.

Bleuler, M. & Bleuler, R. (1935). Rorschach's ink blot test and racial psychology: peculiarities of Moroccans. In *Character and Personality*, **4**, 97–114.

Bleuler, M. (1941). *Krankheitsverlauf, Persönlichkeit und Familienbild Schizophrener und ihre gegenseitigen Beziehungen*. Leipzig: Verlag Georg Thieme.

Bleuler, M. (1941). Das Wesen der Schizophrenieremission nach Schockbehandlung. *Z. ges. Neurol. Psychiat.*, **173**, 553–97.

Bleuler, M. (1943). Die spätschizophrenen Krankheitsbilder. *Fortschr. Neurol. Psychiat.*, **15**, 259–90.

Bleuler, M. (1951). Forschungen und Begriffswandlungen in der Schizophrenielehre 1941–1950. *Fortschr. Neurol. Psychiat.*, **19**, 385–452.

Bleuler, M. (1954). *Endokrinologische Psychiatrie*. Stuttgart: Verlag Thieme.

Bleuler, M. (1955). Familial and personal background of alcoholics. In *Etiology of Chronic Alcoholism*, ed. O. Diethelm, pp. 116–66. Springfield, Illinois: C. C. Thomas.

Bleuler, M. & Stoll, W. (1955). Clinical use of reserpine in psychiatry: comparison with chlorpromazine. *Ann. N. Y. Acad. Sci.*, **61**, 167–73.

Bleuler, M. (1962). Early Swiss sources of Adolf Meyer's concepts. *Am. J. Psychiat.*, **119/3**, 193–6.

Bleuler, M. (1964). Endokrinologische Psychiatrie. In *Psychiatrie der Gegenwart*, vol. I/lb, part B, ed. H. W. Gruhle, R. Jung, W. Mayer-Gross & M. Müller, pp. 160–252. Berlin: Springer.

Bleuler, M., Willi, J. & Bühler, H. R. (1966). *Akute psychische Begleiterschenungen körperlicher Krankheiten, akuter exogener Reaktionstypus*. Stuttgart: Thieme.

Bleuler, M. (1968). A 23-year longitudinal study of 208 schizophrenics and impressions in regard to the nature of schizophrenia. In *Transmission of Schizophrenia*, ed. D. Rosenthal & S. S. Kety, pp. 3–12. Oxford: Pergamon Press.

Bleuler, M. (1972). *Die schizophrenen Geistesstörungen im Lichte langjähriger Kranken – und Familien – Geschichten mit einem Beitrag von A. Uchtenhagen*. Stuttgart: Thieme. 673 pp. (English translation: *Schizophrenic Psychoses*. Yale University Press, 1978.)

Bleuler, M. (1979). Endokrinologische Psychiatrie. In *Psychiatrie der Gegenwart* (2. Auflage), Bd I, ed. K. P. Kisker, J. E. Mayer, C. Müller & E. Strömgren, pp. 257–343. Berlin: Springer.

Bleuler, M. (1979). *Lehrbuch der Psychiatrie von Eugen Bleuler, 7.–14. Auflage 1942–1979, neu bearbeitet von M. Bleuler*. Berlin: Springer.

Bleuler, M. (1979). On schizophrenic psychoses: Adolf Meyer Lecture 1978. *Am. J. Psych.*, **136**, 1403–9.

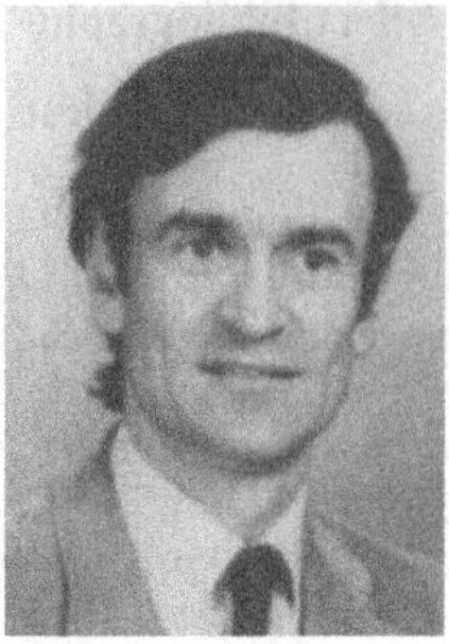

2 · ANTHONY CLARE

I understand that I am likely to be some 20 years younger than most of the other contributors to this volume. This fact makes my position more than usually precarious and cautions prudence in making statements concerning as controversial a subject as the state and future of psychiatry. I am particularly conscious of the fact that whereas others may well consider the subject in the context of a past which they have shared and shaped, I can consider it only from the standpoint of the present and the future. I realise, too, that individuals who are called upon near the end of their professional lives to comment on the achievements and deficiencies of their chosen field of expertise are tempted to draw much comfort, inevitably and understandably, from the fact that whatever its contemporary imperfections, it is a significant advance over what existed even during the recent past. My contribution, therefore, must, of necessity, be a partial one and lack this historical dimension. As against that, however, considerations of the future may have marginally more relevance for me than for many of my fellow contributors, given that, barring any unexpected or premature developments, psychiatric or otherwise, I will have to live through any future that we are invited to consider.

Personal background and professional experience

I was born and raised in Dublin, Ireland, and educated at a Jesuit college. The reputation of that order is somewhat sinister in the English-speaking world, yet in Ireland, the recollections of James Joyce notwithstanding, the Jesuits exert an influence which is largely liberal and benign. It is largely to them, and to one man in particular, that I feel I owe such ideological scepticism and intellectual curiosity as I possess.

It was curiosity, coupled with a desire to do something useful, that drew me into medicine. The same impulses subsequently directed me towards psychiatry as a branch of medicine that promised exciting advances, challenges and possibilities. I also believed that a vigorous and soundly based psychiatry would do much to correct what appeared to me at the time to be a disturbingly excessive organic emphasis within general medicine.

My undergraduate medical training at the beginning of the 1960s at University College, Dublin, differed little, I suspect, from that provided in any of the better-known medical schools in Britain or the United States. Irish surgeons were vigorous teachers, incisive, single-minded and opinionated. Irish physicians were intellectually more fastidious. Both, however, exuded a serene confidence in medicine's achievements. In so far as they regarded psychiatry at all, they did so with disdain, and the contemporary medical view of psychiatrists as 'purveyors of mumbo-jumbo at the worst and of brilliant dialectics at the best' expressed by a leading British professor of medicine would almost certainly have been their own (Peart, 1979).

After interning in a family practice programme in Syracuse, New York, I returned to Dublin to obtain a higher qualification in medicine. I then spent two years in psychiatric training at St Patrick's Hospital in Dublin (founded by Jonathan Swift over 200 years ago), and I then applied to and was accepted by the Maudsley Hospital for further postgraduate training. I started on what seemed to me to be a highly auspicious date, 1 January 1970. Sir Aubrey Lewis, some of whose writings I was already familiar with, had retired some years previously, yet much of what had been initiated during his period as Professor of Psychiatry still operated: most particularly the tutorial system and the three-year M. Phil. degree at the University of London, with its unique integration of clinical training and research work. Indeed, I proved to be one of the last psychiatric trainees to take the qualification, which was unfortunately dropped shortly after the formation of the Royal College of Psychiatrists and the inauguration of that College's membership examination. Such capacity will not be developed by working for the College examination for it contains no serious research component, lacks the close relation to psychiatric training represented by a tutorial approach, promises and subsequently delivers an exceedingly uneven standard and encourages what Lewis termed 'the

DPM outlook' (Lewis, 1947) whereby trainees and teachers alike become preoccupied with syllabuses, cram courses and potted textbooks to the exclusion of studies and work more appropriate to the complex task of psychiatric education. Despite the efforts of a group of my contemporaries to forestall the fledgling College's decision to introduce an examination of this kind (I was the founder Chairman of the Association of Psychiatrists in Training), the membership examination went ahead. It is scant satisfaction that a decade later one sees the gloomy predictions made at that time now fulfilled.

Of those individuals within psychiatry who have influenced me most, Professor Norman Moore, my first mentor, encouraged me to become a psychiatrist; it was he who ascribed considerable importance to the need for a psychiatrist to be first and foremost a competent and well-trained physician. Another influential psychiatrist was Dr F. Kräupl Taylor, for whom I was one of the last Maudsley registrars to work before his retirement and who combined enormous personal flair and genuine wisdom with an authentic eclecticism in his clinical management of patients, an approach which avoided the granting of pre-eminence to biological, psychological, or social approaches. Professor Michael Shepherd has also been a singular influence by virtue of his steadfast commitment to the scientific principles of research and his insistence on the necessity for scrupulous standards of diagnostic practice at a time when diagnosis in psychiatry has been, and indeed still is, being portrayed by some critics as a sterile exercise. For these men I worked as a trainee psychiatrist and their influence was direct and personal. I met Sir Aubrey Lewis only a handful of times, and then fleetingly. I know his views only through his writings, which are his particular legacy to me and, I suspect, to many of my contemporaries. No other psychiatrist in Britain, perhaps in the English-speaking world, has so magisterially and comprehensively reviewed and evaluated the large and intricate issues which split psychiatry, issues such as the definition of mental illness, the mind–body relationship, the position of psychiatry *vis-à-vis* the biological sciences on the one hand and the social and behavioural sciences on the other, the foundations of psychiatric education and training, the role of research and the contribution of the postgraduate institute. It is, of course, true that others have written, and written wisely, on such subjects, but Lewis appears to be seeing them in terms of an overall philosophy of his subject. Where others appear to be part of the game about whose aspects they see fit to comment, Lewis writes from a position of detachment and disinterest and with a panoptic vision of the entire field of play. This is an achievement all the more remarkable given the distaste he shared with Locke for the all-embracing general theory, 'a sort of waking dream with which men have warmed their Heads', and his notable dislike of all-embracing explanations. In the circumstances, I cannot but reflect wryly on the accusation levelled at Lewis, most emphatically by the late Erwin Stengel, that his scepticism and his caution deterred erstwhile psychiatric recruits from entering psychiatry. For my part, I found Lewis's dislike of ideology encouraging and was grateful for his ice-cold candour in admitting to the shortcomings of the subject, an honesty which represented an invigorating alternative to the self-aggrandisment and over-weening confidence that psychiatrists unfortunately appear all too prone to exhibit.

Current status of psychiatry

On completion of my postgraduate training, I was offered a research post in the General Practice Research Unit at the Institute of Psychiatry. I was immediately confronted by a paradox. Psychiatry, as understood within the orthodox psychiatric hospital and as portrayed within the average psychiatric textbook, actually represents less than five per cent of the total amount of psychological and social morbidity coming into contact with the medical services of a country such as Britain. Of the other 95 per cent, psychiatrists have little first-hand knowledge, yet it tends to be psychiatrists who see themselves as the appropriate teachers of those professionals – the general practitioners, the social workers, the health visitors and so on – whose daily work involves them in the identification and treatment of thi enormous burden of sickness. The situation is analogous to that which I had noted as a medical student: confronted by a medical or surgical patient whose depressive or phobic symptoms had been detected, the consultant in a general hospital would decide that such a problem fell within the ambit of his psychiatric colleague, whose familiarity with this type of patient, by contrast with his experience of seriously ill, psychotic patients, was often inadequate. Such a situation has been improved somewhat by the policy of deploying and training psychiatrists in general hospital settings but, of course, they are still seeing the tip of the iceberg, although this is now a general medical iceberg rather than a purely psychiatric one. Nor is this partial view altered by the rotation of general practitioners through six months or more of hospital psychiatry, where they will learn to identify and treat patients whom they will rarely encounter in their own sphere of practice.

Doubtless, the same criticism could be made, and is being made, about hospital medicine, but the issue carries a particular bite and urgency in the case of psychiatry, for it raises the question of what constitutes the core of the discipline. What is it that the psychiatrist is particularly trained to do that distinguishes him from others, such as the GP and the social worker, the counsellor and the priest, whose professional paths so often overlap with his own? Having raised the question, I feel bound to attempt an answer. I see little virtue in, or possibility of, training enough psychiatrists to cope with the psychological and social aspects of primary health care or of medical and surgical conditions which present to our specialist colleagues in their clinics and wards. Strengthening primary health care and general hospital psychiatry will not be achieved by increasing the number of psychiatrists but by educating general practitioners and hospital specialists to recognise that all disorders have a psychological and, indeed, a social as well as a physical dimension.

It has become increasingly evident that the insistence on recruiting, training and deploying more psychiatrists only serves to entrench the incorrigibly dualistic conception of medicine. The very distinction between physical and mental, which is implicit in the designation of psychiatry as a distinct branch of medicine, emphasises the extent to which Cartesian dualism, while publicly disavowed, is embraced in practice. Such a dualism is also detectible within psychiatry itself in the shape of a spurious polarisation between psychological and biological approaches to understanding and treating psychiatric conditions. In Lewis's words, 'If the dualism is denied, then the territory of psychiatry becomes theoretically coextensive with medicine.'

We still find it difficult to speak intelligibly about the pathology of mental disorder except in two languages, the somatic and the psychological. Nowhere is this better illustrated than in the case of schizophrenia, where it does sometimes appear that were a biological factor, such as a pathognomonic enzyme defect or a slow-acting virus to be implicated causally, many psychiatrists would conclude that they no longer had any contribution to make to the diagnosis and treatment of patients with the disorder who should then be handed over to the physicians. Such a view reveals a crude reductionism of Emerson's witty physician who found the creed in the biliary duct and used to affirm that if there was disease in the liver the man became a Calvinist and if that organ was sound he became a Unitarian. This is to misunderstand the nature of the contemporary role of the psychiatrist. At present he is the custodian of the psychological and social dimensions of disease because these have been persistently neglected in the 200 years since the scientific revolution flowered with medicine.

Accordingly, it can be argued that the goal of psychiatrists should not be the preservation of their speciality but rather the re-establishment of the social and psychological perspectives within the heart of medicine itself. This achievement would render the specialty of psychiatry, a speciality hived off from and functioning largely independently of general medicine, virtually redundant.

The contemporary psychiatrist, however, in addition to taking prime responsibility for the diagnosis and treatment of the psychoses and the severe neuroses, is involved within general and primary care medicine. He is also becoming increasingly involved in problems which are by no means his exclusive preserve and which theoretically could be managed by properly trained non-psychiatric and even non-medical personnel. That the psychiatrist has a consulting role to play in the management of such conditions as addictions, alcoholism, and marital and family problems may be reasonable enough, but that he should take over the principal or even a major responsibility is more debatable. Once again, it is a question of balance. Perhaps in the future psychiatrists will still be expected to perform such a consultant role, but in the light of experience that they themselves have acquired as a result of working within the settings of primary care, medical outpatient departments, surgical wards and other places where these problems appear.

One of the more regrettable developments within psychiatry has been its fissiparous tendency. Social psychiatry, for example, which is no more than an emphasis on understanding the interaction between social and clinical events (Wing, 1971), becomes elevated into a specific 'model'. Behavioural approaches, based on some success in the treatment of particular neurotic conditions, form the launching-pad for a determined effort to split psychiatry into two parts, the 'behavioural' part to be managed by clinical psychologists and the 'organic' part to be managed by doctors (Eysenck, 1975). Psychotherapists fight for their own sub-speciality while insisting that their particular approach underpins all aspects of psychiatric theory and practice (Wolff, 1973). The more single-minded biologists treat their patients in a manner indistinguishable from that adopted by the most organically minded physicians in general medicine (Hunter, 1973).

The consequences for psychiatric training, particularly postgraduate training, are serious. In Britain the proliferation of committees and working parties concerned with establishing suitable postgraduate training programmes tends to conceal the extent to which issues, such as registration and accreditation, overshadow certain important questions.

These questions relate to the unattractiveness of psychiatry, the quality of training, the proper balance to be struck between so-called 'general' psychiatry and the proliferating sub-specialties, and the relative importance of personal tuition and clinical apprenticeship compared with the growing emphasis on day-release courses, lectures and packaged cram courses geared towards boards and examinations. It is by no means inevitable that postgraduate psychiatric education will be improved significantly by devising ever-more complicated accreditation procedures and by insisting that trainees spend mandatory periods of time in particular posts. That the quality can be improved is unarguable (indeed, it is imperative), but this will surely require greater attention being devoted to those aspects of training that cultivate a student's capacity to weigh evidence and examine speculations about what Lewis termed 'the intangible material of psychiatry which can be much more elusive and deceptive than somatic phenomena'.

It is important that any critical evaluation of the state of psychiatry should take account of the achievements and possibilities. In the 15 years or so that I have been a psychiatrist there has been progress, although no advance to match the developments in the pharmacological treatment of psychiatric morbidity of the previous decade. Our understanding of neuronal function and transmission is evolving, albeit slowly, towards an appropriate level of sophistication. There has been a considerable clarification of the relative role of genetic, social and environmental factors in schizophrenia, affective disorders and, to a lesser extent, alcoholism. Epidemiological research has illuminated the nature and natural history of those ubiquitous psychological and social disorders which constitute the greater portion of psychiatric morbidity in the community. The development of novel techniques of behavioural modification for the relief of crippling anxiety, obsessive–compulsive disorders and phobias represents a genuine, although modest, advance. There have been exciting developments in neuropsychology in relation to our understanding of hemispheric function and memory and, more tentatively, to our knowledge of limbic system function. More disappointing has been the relative failure to advance knowledge of the efficacy of psychotherapy. Such research as has been conducted (Hogan, 1979) lends scant support to those who argue the case for psychoanalysis and psychoanalytically derived psychotherapy.

In practice, psychoanalysis, the most time-consuming, expensive and complicated of the psychotherapies, is reserved for those who are minimally ill or, indeed, who are not ill at all. This is a remarkable transposition of the more familiar situation in medicine wherein the most complex treatment is reserved for the most afflicted patient. The suggestion that such elements as are therapeutic in psychotherapy are common to a variety of psychological interventions, including behavioural approaches, and do not include transference analysis, dynamic interpretation and the other definitive characteristics of classical psychoanalysis has important implications for the development and organisation of psychiatric and medical services, to say nothing of psychiatric and general medical training.

Future prospects of psychiatry

If psychiatry can avoid further fragmentation into sub-specialities, each struggling for pre-eminence, each claiming a definitive role, each competing for meagre resources, then such progress as has been made may be sustained. For once, economic reality may combine with theoretical wisdom to produce a realistic and pragmatic psychiatry capable of integrating within a medicine that has likewise evolved from its currently excessive organic orientation. Should the idea of psychiatry metamorphosing back into psychological medicine dismay sociologists, psychologists, anthropologists and related behavioural and social scientists currently working in the general area of mental health, they might reflect that such an integration, if enacted with prudence and generosity, promises not merely a greater recognition of psychological and social contributions to the understanding of medical conditions but a more significant role for all of these sciences in this process than has been achieved to date.

At the same time I am fully aware of the siren voices tempting psychiatry to move in two opposing directions. One is the voice of biology, which has acquired new authority, partly through such exciting developments as the discovery of the endorphins and partly through a disenchantment with the social sciences – a disenchantment, it should be said, which owes something to the over-enthusiastic and excessive claims made in that direction. The other is a voice hostile to medicine. This voice preaches 'holism' and beckons psychiatry out into the soft, doughy arena of gestalt psychology and encounter therapy to minister to the needs of people less ill than dissatisfied and more appropriately classified as demoralised than disordered. A retreat by psychiatry into the pit of reductionist, technological and blinkered organic science from which general medicine is currently struggling to emerge would prove disastrous for the future not merely of psychiatry but of medicine itself. The further dilution of psychiatric theory by the woollier formulations of fringe psychotherapy would spell doom for psychiatry's efforts to establish for itself a sound foundation in the basic biological as well as social sciences.

The future of psychological medicine will depend on there being available individuals capable of standing above the fierce battle for research monies, the seductive temptations of psychiatric expansionism and the immediate gratification provided by short-lived and spurious breakthroughs. Psychiatry will be pushed, as it has been pushed in the past, by political and administrative as well as by scientific and educational forces. It still lacks the comprehensive security of a scientifically established foundation similar to that provided by the physical systems of the body in medicine, and this lack makes it especially vulnerable to the various winds of ideological fashion that blow around it.

For this reason, over and above many others, I hold firmly to the conviction that the future of psychological medicine stands or falls on the extent to which it establishes its scientific status, using the Platonic definition of science as the discovery of things as they really are. At present there is a movement to disparage science for its alleged ability to measure only the trivial; the immeasurable and the important are said to be above the mundane limits of scientific enquiry. It is fashionable too to portray science as itself a pliable philosophy penetrated by the political heritage and social values of its time. Yet it was a psychiatrist and philosopher who observed that 'the true measure for scientific investigation must always be the substantial fact, valid and enduring' (Jaspers, 1923), and it is salutary to note that the closing pages of that majestic book has Karl Jaspers pondering the catastrophe for psychiatry should it ever depart from its search for a scientific foundation.

Questions and answers

1. You say that you envisage psychiatry becoming 'virtually redundant' in time. What, if any, would then be the functions of the psychiatrist?

The reintegration of psychiatry within the mainstream of medicine requires that psychiatrists reassume their medical roles (Eisenberg, 1979). As a separate speciality, psychiatry drifts from one meretricious explanatory theory to another, ready prey for the competing ideologies that flourish in the wasteland which lies between the biological and social sciences (Clare, 1980). Despite the confident assertions of so many psychiatrists, the theoretical and clinical foundations of the subject remain remarkably unsound and ill-suited to the pretentious edifices erected over them. While differences between doctors are expressed within a context of commonly shared assumptions and certainties concerning the underlying biological nature of the human organism, psychiatrists differ over the very nature of mental disorder itself. Some even doubt its existence.

In the circumstances, to conclude that the neurobiological basis of psychiatric practice is becoming a reality (Guze, 1978) seems a trifle premature, but I have little doubt that the main impetus should be, and arguably is, in that direction. But if this is indeed so, and if psychiatry is moving back to its medical origins, becoming psychological medicine once again, then what becomes of the psychiatrist? For as far into the future as one dare peer, the diagnosis and treatment of serious psychotic illness seems likely to remain the prime responsibility of the specialist in disturbed mental functioning. But is there anything left? If the growing infiltration of the undergraduate medical schools by clinical and academic psychiatrists, the growing collaboration between psychiatrists and general practitioners (Clare & Williams, 1979) and the burgeoning popularity of what is termed 'liaison psychiatry' are to match the expectations placed on them by their more enthusiastic protagonists, then surely tomorrow's physicians, surgeons, gynaecologists, paediatricians and, most particularly, general practitioners are going to prove more accomplished in the task of integrating somatic and psychological manifestations of ill-health? If, however, such progress remains elusive, and if the medical schools and general hospitals revert to or persist in a policy whereby the model of human functioning held up to the student is 'a machine, a physicochemical arrangement of prefabricated, predetermined parts which work like a computor tied to a pump and stove' (Barzun, 1973), the psychiatrists, whether they remain separate specialists or not, will have failed. Either way, the role of psychiatrist as psychiatrist seems likely to be severely circumscribed. Nor can psychiatrists seek a new justification for their existence by moving away from psychological medicine and into areas already occupied by or being invaded steadily by professionals from non-medical disciplines, who claim, with some justification, that their interventions are more effective, more economic and more acceptable.

The growing popularity for programmes wherein the psychiatrist works alongside his general medical and primary care colleagues has implications not merely for the future clinical shape and practice of psychological medicine but for biomedical research in general. Isolated in his mental hospital and catchment area service, the clinical psychiatrist currently continues to be 'a consumer rather than a producer of research' (Shepherd,

1981). Alongside his medical colleagues, and more particularly his colleagues in the basic biological and behavioural sciences, the psychiatrist would be and is better placed to make a particular contribution to advancing the frontiers of knowledge concerning the nature and extent of disease in general, and the malfunctioning brain and central nervous system in particular.

Of course there are hazards. Anyone familiar with the difficulties encountered by the fledgling speciality of psychiatry as it struggled in the shadow of the prestigious medical specialities cannot contemplate the notion of a reabsorption of psychiatry within medicine with equanimity. It may well be that psychiatry will not survive at all and that any attempt to widen the perspective and the horizons of medicine to take into account not merely the psychological aspects of illness but also its behavioural manifestations, social epidemiology and cultural significance will falter in the face of an insistent and confident biological and technological reductionism. If psychiatry attempts the re-integration advocated by Eisenberg it may lose everything. But if it does not attempt it, and if it stubbornly remains a separate speciality, an anachronistic concrete expression of Cartesian dualism, then it will lose everything.

2. What are the 'implications' to which you refer on page 21?

The demonstration of a large pool of psychiatric morbidity within the community (Shepherd, Cooper, Brown & Kalton, 1966) has led some to argue for a dramatic expansion in the availability and the number of psychotherapists. Yet there is precious little evidence that psychotherapy, in its classical analytical forms, can be applied to the realities of primary health and general medical care. There have been various modifications attempted to meet the needs and demands of patients presenting to general medical and primary care services but the net result has been the evolution of a psychotherapy which amounts to little more than 'steady support, a sympathetic understanding attitude, a sophisticated understanding of the complexities of human behaviour, and at best a certain wisdom about life' (Madden, 1979). Not unreasonably, Madden concludes that such non-specific features should be part and parcel of all patient care and hardly justify the elaborate edifice of a metapsychology. Such studies of the efficacy of psychotherapy as have been performed tend to support such a view (Truax & Mitchell, 1972; Lieberman, Yalon & Miles, 1973; Sloane, Staples, Cristol, Yorkston & Whipple, 1975; Luborsky, Singer & Luborsky 1975; Glass 1976). Indeed, the work of Sloane and his colleagues, showing as it did the relatively modest gains derived by formal psychotherapy and behavioural approaches over fairly basic intervention, serves to emphasise the need to identify what precisely it is that is specific to psychotherapy. The equivalent recorded improvement of the controls in their work, social and overall adjustment, indicates the extent to which improvement may be achieved with therapeutic approaches which are far less complicated, opaque, time-consuming and expensive than psychotherapy. These are precisely the sort of questions of psychiatry. The financing, organisation and delivery of health care in these settings tolerate time-consuming and expensive treatments of unproven worth less patiently than psychiatry tolerates them. Yet another of the benefits which might be expected to accrue from the close relationship between psychiatry and the rest of medicine is a more severe scrutiny of the therapeutic strategies deployed throughout both.

3. In view of your interest in and your strictures on the education of psychiatrists, would you comment on the sharp decline in recruitment of the speciality over the past few years?

An overall decline in recruitment almost certainly has more than one underlying cause. Psychiatric recruitment has declined in Britain and the United States as general practice has expanded and it is difficult to avoid the conclusion that the two trends are interrelated. The increased prestige of general practice within general medicine contrasts favourably with the persistently low image of psychiatry within medicine and within those behavioural and social sciences with which psychiatry has everyday dealings. Improved organisation and working conditions, together with the long-standing 'holistic' emphasis of general practice, have also contributed to the resurgence of primary care at a time when vogues for 'person-centred' health care, prevention and multidisciplinary team approaches hold sway. Psychiatry lacks the theoretical clarity and technical confidence of general medicine and the opportunities for and satisfactions derived from the provision of comprehensive medical care that is the hallmark of good general practice.

It is tempting, no doubt, to seek the explanations for the fall in recruitment in terms of the scientific biases of the students or, more particularly, of those who select them for admission into medical school. But such an explanation lives uneasily with the healthy recruitment of graduates into general practice. In the circumstances, it is difficult to avoid placing some of the responsibility for the failure to recruit more and better young doctors into psychiatry at the feet of those whose responsibility it is to teach them psychiatry in medical school. Students emulate those teachers they respect. In this way, careers in research as well as in clinical practice are stimulated. In this regard, it is surprising to note that one study of newly recruited British psychiatrists revealed that, for the great majority, contact with psychiatric teachers both before and after medical graduation had been of secondary importance or of no importance at all in affecting the choice of psychiatry as a career; the prospective psychiatrist's own curiosity about people and his view of psychiatry as an important and interesting branch of medicine were of much greater importance (Brook, 1973). Around the same time as Brook was publishing his findings, an American psychiatrist was predicting confidently that there would always be a place for psychiatrists 'because collectively we belong to the only field concerned with the whole person' (Grinker, 1975). However, from the vantage-point of the early 1980s, it is not at all so obvious that curiosity in people and concern for the whole person can be successfully sustained only by embarking on a psychiatric career.

Finally, there are signs that psychiatry in recent years may have overemphasised the importance of training programmes, rotational schemes and accreditation exercises at the expense of the clinical apprenticeship, individual supervision and research undertaken in the clinical setting. Many psychiatrists engage in little teaching and undertake no research. Not surprisingly, many junior psychiatrists follow their example. The impact on morale, vitality and confidence of the speciality is reflected in recruitment. Training programmes can be elaborated, goals enumerated, objectives codified and standards set and for a brief heady period we can pretend that such exercises represent the development of the speciality rather than merely aspirations relating to it. But reality cannot be thwarted for long. For all the efforts and energies devoted to establishing respectable educational programmes, the fact remains that a very small proportion of medical graduates came forward to participate in them. And it is difficult to resist the conclusion that one reason for this paucity of recruits is the fact that the impact of the individual psychiatrist on potential recruits is either non-existent or negative. I have testified to the positive influence of particular individuals in my own choice of a career in psychiatry and my subsequent progress within it. I may be exaggerating from the basis of personal experience, yet it is difficult to avoid the conclusion that psychiatry in recent years may have lost some of its appeal to the newly qualified doctor because psychiatrists have tended to neglect the personal aspects of psychiatric education, training, clinical practice and research in favour of more impersonal ones, a mistake which general practice, for example, by virtue of its strong clinical roots and emphasis, has not yet emulated.

References

Barzun, J. (1973). The education of candidates for medical school. *Bulletin of the New York Academy of Medicine*, **49**, 253–7.

Brook, P. (1973). *Psychiatrists in Training*. British Journal of Psychiatry: Special Publication No. 7. Ashford, Kent: Headley Brothers.

Clare, A. W. (1980). *Psychiatry in Dissent* (2nd edition). London: Tavistock.

Clare, A. W. & Williams, P. (1979). Future trends in research into primary care psychiatry. In *Psychosocial Disorders in General Practice*, pp. 325–32, ed. P. Williams & A. Clare. London: Academic Press.

Eisenberg, L. (1979). Interface between medicine and psychiatry. *Comprehensive Psychiatry*, **20**, 1, 1–14.

Eysenck, H. J. (1975). *The Future of Psychiatry*. London: Methuen.

Glass, G. V. (1976). 'Primary, secondary and meta-analysis of research.' Paper presented as presidential address to the 1976 Journal Meeting of the American Educational Research Association, San Francisco, 4 April 1976.

Grinker, R. R. (1975). The future educational needs of psychiatrists. *American Journal of Psychiatry*, **132**, 3, 259–62.

Guze, S. B. (1978). Nature of psychiatric illness: why psychiatry is a branch of medicine. *Comprehensive Psychiatry*, **19**, 4, 295–307.

Hogan, D. B. (1979). *The Regulation of Psychotherapists. Vol. I. A Study in the Philosophy and Practice of Professional Regulation*. Cambridge, Mass: Ballinger.

Hunter, R. (1973). Psychiatry and neurology: psychosyndrome or brain disease? *Proceedings of the Royal Society of Medicine*, **66**, 17–22.

Jaspers, K. (1923). *General Psychopathology*. English translation: J. Hoenig & M. W. Hamilton. Manchester University Press, 1963.

Lewis, A. (1947). The education of psychiatrists. *Lancet* ii, 79–83.

Lieberman, M. A., Yalon, I. D. & Miles, M. B. (1973). *Encounter Groups: First Facts*. New York: Basic Books.

Luborsky, L., Singer, B. & Luborsky, L. (1975). Comparative studies of psychotherapies: Is it true that everyone has won and all must have prizes? *Archives of General Psychiatry*, **32**, 995–1008.

Madden, T. A. (1979). The doctors, the patients and their care: Balint reassessed. *Psychological Medicine*, **9**, 5–8.

Peart, W. S. (1979). Research in psychiatry: a view from general medicine. *Psychological Medicine*, **9**, 205–6.

Shepherd, M. (1981). Psychiatric research in medical perspective. *British Medical Journal*, **282**, 961–3.

Shepherd, M., Cooper, B., Brown, A. C. & Kalton, G. W. (1966). *Psychiatric Illness in General Practice*. London: Oxford University Press.

Sloane, R. B., Staples, F. R., Cristol, A. H., Yorkston, N.J. & Whipple, K. (1975). *Psychotherapy vs. Behaviour Therapy*. Cambridge, Mass.: Harvard University Press.

Truax, C. B. & Mitchell, K. M. (1972). Research on certain therapist interpersonal skills in relation to progress and outcome. In *Handbook of Psychotherapy and Behavioural Change*, ed. A. E. Bergin & S. L. Garfield. New York: Wiley.

Wing, J. K. (1971). Social psychiatry. *British Journal of Hospital Medicine*, 5, 53–6.

Wolff, H. H. (1973). The place of psychotherapy in the district psychiatric services. In *Policy For Action*, pp. 117–28, ed. R.H. Cawley & G. McLachlan. Nuffield Provincial Hospitals Trust and Oxford University Press.

Select bibliography

Clare, A.W. (1971). The training of psychiatrists. *Lancet*, ii, 753–6.

Clare, A. W. (1976). *Psychiatry in Dissent.* Controversial Issues in Contemporary Psychiatry. London: Tavistock, and Philadelphia: Institute for the Study of Public Issues (2nd edition 1980).

Clare, A. W. & Cairnes, V. E. (1978). Design, development and use of standardised interview to assess social maladjustment and dysfunction in community studies. *Psychological Medicine*, 8, 589–604.

Clare, A.W. & Shepherd, M. (1978). Psychiatry and family medicine. In *Scientific Foundations of Family Medicine*, pp. 105–23, ed. J. Fry, E. Gambrill & R. Smith. London: Heinemann.

Clare, A. W. (1979). Psychiatric and social aspects of premenstrual complaints in women attending general practitioners. In *Emotion and Reproduction*, pp. 177–84, ed. L. Carenza & L. Zichella. London & New York: Academic Press.

Clare, A. W. (1979). Brief psychotherapy: new approaches. In *Symposium on Brief Psychotherapy*, pp. 93–109, R. B. Sloan & F. Staples. Psychiatric Clinics of North America. Philadelphia: W. B. Saunders.

Clare, A. W. (1979). The disease concept in psychiatry. In *Essentials of Postgraduate Psychiatry*, ed. P. Hill, R. Murray & A. Thorley, chapter 3, pp. 56–76. London & New York: Academic Press.

Clare, A. W. & Davies, G. (1979). Psychiatry in general practice. In *Essentials of Postgraduate Psychiatry*, ed. P. Hill, R. Murray & A. Thorley, chapter 17, pp. 567–98. London & New York: Academic Press.

Williams, P. & Clare, A. Editors (1979). *Psychosocial Disorders in General Practice.* London & New York: Academic Press.

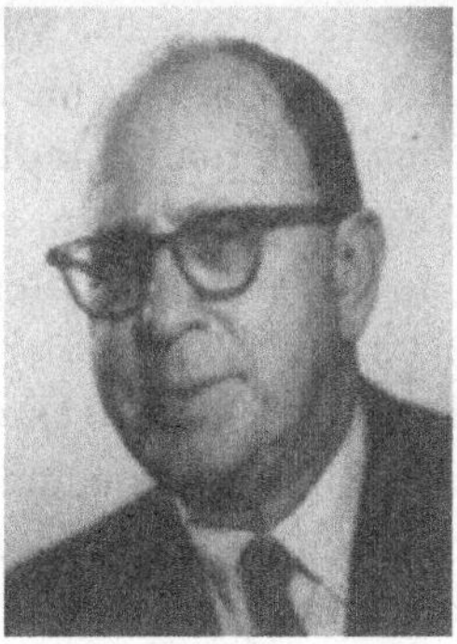

3 · ROY R. GRINKER Sr

Personal background and professional experience

Born in 1900 I was the first child of my parents, and the first grandchild in the family, thereby receiving considerable attention and affection, but I was also the focus of great expectations. My father's intellectual orientation as well as his profession of neuropsychiatry surrounded me with books, which I read voraciously on the floor of the library. In fact, wherever I studied abroad later, I literally devoured the professor's books. The Grinker genes, as far as I can trace them (although the beginnings of the name are unknown), started with a Grinker schoolteacher, who was a member of the Rothschild colony in Palestine and remained there when the colony failed.

Grinkers were subsequently scattered, although in small numbers, in Israel, Africa, South America and in many cities in the United States, pursuing professional careers in medicine, law and engineering. There was no question but that I was expected to follow my father's model and that of his favourite pupil, Percival Bailey, although the repeated statement, 'You will be better than I', became a 'monkey on my back' and the source of much depression.

I was the silent listener and observer at the weekly family dinner and post-prandial discussions. But also, during Sunday walks in the park, when my father made rounds on patients in 'rest-cures', he taught me how to observe and to describe, and he emphasised the crime of exaggeration. At the evening meal he described patients whom he had examined that day, expecting me to make a diagnosis, which my mother always volunteered first as 'syphilis', a warning to me about the dangers of sex. Another competitor was my maternal grandfather, who gave me an allowance of 25 cents weekly if I promised to become an architect. This probably had something to do with my later planning a psychiatric institute and clinic.

My extensive childhood reading led me to experiment with imaginative writing, for which I received commendation and encouragement from my teachers, and I later went on to publish some of my work. But my first language was German, and I only changed to English when my father spent a solitary year studying neurology abroad. For many years (and often now) I found my sentences containing many qualifying clauses, and the verbs wandering to the end of some sentences. Yet in college my English professor awarded me a grade A without reading my examination paper.

Although I had fun playing with other children and was moderately skilled in tennis, my greatest pleasure was derived from reading and thinking. Indeed, I could do little else with a congenital weakness in my back muscles, colour blindness, and tone deafness; it was a struggle to overcome these handicaps.

During my medical school days psychiatry was taught badly, if at all, and neurology was little better. My teacher in psychiatry, a bitter bachelor, taught by reading chapters from Kraepelin's textbook in a droning voice that promptly lulled me to sleep. I vowed then that I would never be a psychiatrist. My decision was reinforced by attending conferences as an intern, where the psychiatrists seemed as confused as the patients and were concerned only with problems of legal commitment. Diagnostic conclusions were based on criteria that I could not understand.

My father furnished me with funds for a postgraduate year abroad, and I combined a honeymoon and education in Vienna in Marburg's laboratory, in Zurich with Von Monakow, in Hamburg with Alfons Jakob, and in London, at Queen's Square, mostly with Gordon Holmes. I certainly learned much neurology but little psychiatry, except for weekly clinics with Eugen Bleuler at Burghölzli, near Zurich. I was happy to work with Holmes but horrified when, after a thorough examination, he kicked his neurotic patients in the buttocks, saying, 'There's nothing the matter with you. Go home and forget it.'

On my return to Chicago I was dedicated to neurology and unhappy with my father's psychotherapy of support, direction, education and suggestion that required weekly visits. He had supported Ernest Jones' paper on psychoanalysis in Chicago in 1912, but became unhappy by his patients' transferences. As a result, he could not support my attempts in Zurich to join David Levy in analysis with Oberholzer. So, after my father's death and at the invitation of the Dean of the University of Chicago Medical School, I joined that faculty as a neurologist. The university had no psychiatry department, and during an unhappy period working with Percival Bailey, then a neurosurgeon, I was asked to take a two-year Rockefeller Fellowship abroad and to return and start a Department of Psychiatry. Before leaving, I published my textbook, *Neurology*, now in its seventh edition and totally re-written in 1977 by N. Vick. After much discussion and contrary advice, I decided to begin my psychiatric training with an analysis by Sigmund Freud, which angered Critchley and Carmichael, the house officers during the time I clerked at Queen's Square. I later journeyed around the universities in Germany, and finally worked for a time at the Maudsley Hospital, where I enjoyed the contact I had with Aubrey Lewis. On my return to Chicago I found that the university was not ready for psychiatry, which was not, in fact, accepted for another 30 years. I returned, by invitation, to the Michael Reese Hospital, where I have remained for the ensuing 40 years, eventually developing an Institute and a Clinic.

The Second World War intervened, and I knew that I had to participate overseas. I was sent to North Africa, where John Spiegel and I worked together to produce *Men Under Stress*, soon to be reprinted for the third time. The war experience, mostly psychiatric, was the catalyst that solidified my interest in combining psychiatry with organic medicine under the title of 'psychosomatics'.

Current status of psychiatry

It is difficult to discuss psychiatry in terms of current status because of its changing character. At various times I have stated expansively that 'psychiatry is as broad as life', and that 'psychiatry rides madly in all directions'. In fact, the definition of psychiatry has never been so difficult since the time of Kraepelin's medical model, his outcome predictions and the cellular neuropathology of Nissl and Alzheimer. The terminology and conceptual problems that Spitzer has attacked courageously in the third edition of the American Psychiatric Association's Diagnostic and Statistical Manual indicate the perversity of definition in the field.

After my return from military service I began my work on the stress effects of anxiety, anger and depression. It took a decade before a large multidisciplinary team could be sure that Alexander's emotional specificity did not hold. Only in the case of anger could an increase in blood pressure be predicted. For the most part it turned out that specificity was limited to the area of response, since any meaningful stress-stimulus evokes the same stress-response.

Although some theorists have contended that there is only one mental illness, and others that mental illness is a myth promulgated by sadistic psychiatrists in an effort to control others, our task continues to be the construction of a diagnostic differentiation leading to appropriate treatment. There seem to be three main areas: (a) neuroses, (b) personality or character disorders, and (c) psychoses. Neuroses are basically defenses against anxiety; psychoses are genetic–environmental diatheses; and the personality disorders have still to be well-defined.

All psychiatric disorders certainly create problems of living but the questions, 'What', 'How' and 'Why' are only vaguely formulated. In fact, the end results are rapidly changing. Histrionic, dramatic psychoses – for example manics, catatonics and hebephrenics – are now rare. Instead, constricted and restricted personality deviations are on the increase but not as manifestations of one disease.

What we need now are the exact and specific diagnostic criteria so strongly opposed by those non-scientific discussions of psychoanalysts who contend that 'our science' is concerned, by right, only with 'my individual patient'. To ensure some degree of competence in diagnosis, we need methods of observation, verbal information and psychological test data to develop syndromes that include pathognomonic symptoms and exclude defensive and substitute peripheral symptoms.

What we hear repetitively are the statements that depth investigations produce insight. We do not know the meaning of insight; however, we have been able to translate ego functions (seven in all) into five categories of behaviour. In that sense, all of psychiatry is a behavioural science, whether individual patients respond to words or physical tactics. Insight begins when behavioural changes feed back into the psychic apparatus and modify thinking and feeling.

A recent study of differences among psychiatrists from various nations has indicated that the British diagnose manic depression ten times more frequently than the Americans, who specify schizophrenia more frequently. As a result, a subtle change has become evident among the Americans, who now use standard tests for affective disorders (SAD), thereby decreasing the schizophrenic diagnosis. They even doubt now that what we call 'acute schizophrenia' or 'schizoaffective disorders' belong to the large category of the schizophrenias.

Americans constitute a fashion-ridden, unstable society, even in the field of their scientific interests. Thus, the publications on the borderline syndrome, the narcissistic neuroses and psychoses as well as the spectrum concepts have spread rapidly, without concern for significant and empirical research. It is interesting that discursive writing rather than observational data dominates most of our psychiatric periodicals. Hardly a publication contains one third of plausible information. For example, the spectrum concept has overpowered us. The schizophrenic spectrum in the families includes, according to their users, 'acute schizophrenia, pseudoneurotic schizophrenia and the borderline'. However, this view does not accord with acceptable definitions. One may just as well state that schizophrenics, as well as borderlines, arise from 'sick families', which is a meaningless term. Likewise, the depressed syndrome has been associated with a spectrum in the families of origin, consisting of 'colour blindness, blood dyscrasia, alcoholism and asocial behaviour'. Obviously, the diagnosis of the components of the so-called spectrum would require rigorous definition based on careful clinical research.

How do we educate the young psychiatrist? Research models exist, of course, but there are very few of them. Too frequently investigators are reductionists or humanists maintaining a consistency that can be termed bias. Most thinking, in fact, consists of dichotomies. To offset this grievous fault, we need an overall inclusive theoretical base, consisting of a unified theory or what is more generally termed 'general systems theory'. This contains parts related to various part-functions linked to various specific disciplines and integrated by some supraordinate control or regulation. Without such a theoretical approach, properly used, we are destined to remain theoretical partisans. Unfortunately, there are only a few psychiatrists who have sufficient information concerning the wide extent of the parts of the system.

During the years of my psychiatric research, not including my neurological work, I have worked on various subjects, using methods seemingly most appropriate for each. These include systems theory, changes in medical education, psychosomatic research, anxiety and stress, classification of emotional experiences, muscle tension, transactional psychotherapy (not Berne's type), psychiatric social work, classification and subcategories of depression, the borderline syndromes, the borderline patient, schizophrenia, hypothalamic functions, war neuroses (predisposition, stress tolerance test, brief therapy, etc.), identification and normality (homoclites). This work has been published in some 265 papers and 18 books. In addition, I have trained chairmen of departments and various professional ranks in American medical schools.

For almost two decades I was associated with the Archives published by the American Medical Association. For 10 years prior to 1 January, 1970 I was Editor-in-Chief of the *Archives of General Psychiatry*. The following is an excerpt from a note that I published in Volume 1.

> An important reason for the establishment of a new Archives devoted entirely to psychiatry is the realistic recognition that neuropsychiatry has become separated into neurology and psychiatry as distinct clinical specialities. Each group of specialists has been penalized by receiving an *Archives of Neurology and Psychiatry*, of which only half interests it. Although it is true that the structure, function, and pathology of the central nervous system are significant aspects of the basic sciences necessary for the training and development of the broadly educated psychiatrist, the details of existing clinical neurological knowledge are of little interest or practical use, and are not remembered. It is, instead, the extrapolated broad principles that are of importance for the congruence of physiological and psychological functions. Certainly, the psychiatrist should read and understand current research leading to breakthroughs of existing barriers to proper understanding and treatment of the major psychoses, such as newer psychopharmacology, as well as the selected basic advances in neurophysiology significant for the understanding of psychodynamics and psychopathology. These works we shall continue to publish.
>
> We shall publish contributions from all disciplines, whether morphological, physiological, biochemical, endocrinological, psychosomatic, psychological, psychiatric, child-psychiatric, psychoanalytical, sociological, or anthropological, that are related to the study of the behavior of Man in health and illness. We shall attempt to implement the concept that Man's behavior cannot in our day be viewed profitably from a narrow frame of reference. Instead, it requires a broad vision of a totally integrated field composed of many part functions and transactions, which constitute the focus of a wide variety of scientific disciplines. Eventually, a *unified science of behavior* may emerge.
>
> From the time of its inception, the *Archives* recognized that psychiatrists rarely carry on clinical research in isolation, but cooperate with psychologists, social workers, and other social

scientists. A vast number of non-medical disciplines not only learn about personality and its disorders from psychiatrists, but also, in turn, contribute greatly to advances in psychiatric knowledge. The psychiatric field is increasing constantly in breadth and depth, and it needs a forum for the many life disciplines that are concerned with its progress.

Future prospects of psychiatry

The golden era of psychiatry, from the end of World War II to the early 1970s, is no longer with us. The interest in support of the field taken over by the government from the private sector of philanthropists has passed as government grants have dried up. Given that these contained a considerable amount of water, the regulatory bodies and bureaucrats have been difficult to deal with. In fact, a whole new profession of psychopolitics has thrived. Psychosocial etiology has created family research, and the theory that genetic patterns can be altered by psychotherapy, although worth investigating, has created a series of discursive productions called sociobiology. These are interesting, indeed, but without proven value.

In a cartoon by Mel, the teacher is explaining to future doctors of America how one struggled to maintain current knowledge by Continuing Medical Education programmes and examinations. Ira asks, with child-like curiosity, 'And if we flunk, will they demote us to psychiatrists?' Indeed, psychiatry is surrounded by enemies: encounter groups, lay therapists, clinical psychologists and nurse specialists. Everyone wants to get into the therapeutic act, but few want to do research or teach imaginatively. Power is the word in community psychiatry!

The future of psychiatry obviously depends on the development of research in the field, which sadly needs intensive investigation. However, increased knowledge in the field of psychiatry can only be achieved through increased sophistication in research designs and in theoretical concepts. There is no longer room for superficial correlations which have satisfied us until now. Indeed, the complications are so great that young persons interested in investigative careers are often turned aside when they contemplate the intricacies of working in a field concerned with human mentation and behaviour. The complications of human personalities, their high degree of variability and the tremendous difficulties in holding parameters constant understandably induce considerable frustration.

To begin with, it becomes necessary to define what we mean by psychiatry. The older definition took psychiatry to be a medical specialty concerned with clinical phenomena; that is, with the prevention, diagnosis and treatment of mental disturbances. Yet, although the function of a medical psychiatrist is to treat patients, we find that there is no sound knowledge concerning what kind of treatment applied to what kind of patient by what kind of person and in what circumstances achieves what kind of results. This old 'what' question exists despite the fact that many so-called 'helping professions' may achieve some results, but we are in no way clear as to the nature of the causes of the results which satisfy the therapist. The common factor to which we may attribute constructive results may be contact with an understanding, empathic human being for variable periods of time, with opportunities for ventilation of feelings and understanding, if not explanation, by the therapist.

It is in the field of treatment that my own resistances have a high titre, since there are so many possibilities of evaluating results that escape our capability for measurement. Thus, unless one is willing to work for decades within a single area, it may be wiser not to begin.

The newer concept of psychiatry as a conglomeration of contributory sciences obviously predicates that advances will depend on advances in those constituent sciences. This newer definition of psychiatry – and one should use the term scientific psychiatry – really applies to its parts and is opposed to the empirical, impressionistic, prejudged and bias-loaded aspects of medical psychiatry.

If we look at the vast area which psychiatry now covers without even being able to guess how much further it will extend – since psychiatry seems to be 'as broad as life itself' – we find four major divisions that are based on a number of points of view or orientations. First, we can easily recognise the sub-divisions of age which partition psychiatry into more aspects concerned with children, adolescents, adults and the aging. Second, some frames of reference are problem-oriented, such as disease classifications, behavioural manifestations and dynamic or psychoanalytic concepts. These are three approaches which deal with specific problems from separate frames of reference. Third is the action-oriented psychiatry, which is concerned with the study of epidemiology and social engineering and which has as its prime purpose the changing of society so that its citizens will not suffer from frustrations and conflicts that end in sickness. Finally, there is an approach-oriented psychiatry, which can be subdivided into biological, psychological and social. Sometimes these are linked together in one biopsychosocial approach.

The variety of these dimensions has often expressed itself in a conflict of the either/or type; this is resolved sometimes by the adoption of a reductionistic frame of reference and sometimes by a humanistic frame of reference, indicating that such polarities are considered to be quite separate. On the other hand, some attempt has been made to resolve conflicts of this nature by the development of general or unified theories, of which general systems theory is one, and of transactionalism, either as a part of it or another theory. These global theories, however, require many operations and often serve as escape hatches when not synthesised. My own goal of synthesis, based on my neurological background and my dynamic training in psychiatry, led me to become deeply involved in the psychosomatic field.

Turning now to some previous and current so-called breakthroughs which are considered advances in the field, we can see that some have passed their most productive periods, others still are fruitful and some are in the stage of formulation.

At the time of its heyday in the United States, psychoanalysis was considered to be the answer to all the problems of mankind. As a humanistic theory concerned with meanings, it failed to achieve the level required of a science, even though its supporters frequently spoke of 'our science'.

The psychosomatic concept of differentiation points to the need for a full investigation of personality types involved in either the cause, course or results of specific chronic diseases. There is a great deal of work being done which is not necessarily entirely psychological but is of importance in determining differences among people who suffer from chronic degenerative diseases.

The next important breakthrough came through the discovery of psychotherapeutic drugs. The importance of these discoveries lay not only in the fact that certain drugs may decrease activity, excitement and anxiety and that others alleviate depression, but also because of the great stimulus that they provided for the study of specific pharmacology of brain functions in various areas. This paradigm, which is still being developed, leads us to believe that many portions of the brain, with discrete functions contributing to the mosaic of behaviour, may have specific chemical constituents which become disordered and may point the way to specific therapeutic agents. I look forward to great accomplishments in this field of neuropharmacology.

The concept of prevention in the framework of medical psychiatry has moved on to what might be called social psychiatry, which is action-oriented. It conceives of the possibility that if we can shift community functions to develop societies in which frustration, conflict and aggression are lessened, we may prevent mental illness. This pious hope has been confused with community psychiatry, which is really a delivery system concerned with the organisation of facilities. Social psychiatry is a different field: it is one which has not yet developed a paradigm, it has not developed research designs and it has not yet conceived of techniques for evaluation. Whether this field will be productive or not, one cannot tell; but I believe that the role of psychiatry is secondary to it. The sociologists, anthropologists and epidemiologists are primarily concerned with action, viewing the psychiatrist as a consultant and as a person who sets some limiting factors to wild social theories.

Contributing sciences may include biogenetics, anatomy, physiology, biochemistry and many others. Each of these contributing sciences has its own paradigm and can well be applied to attacks on various mental phenomena. There is some hope that the study of evoked potentials and other EEG phenomena will develop some discriminatory analyses of behavioural functions. The immunological aspects of disease may be applied to certain disturbances in the central nervous system that may be due to auto-immunity phenomena. It is certain that the studies of sleep, dreams and also hypnosis may contribute a great deal to the phenomena of aberrant kinds of thinking and behaviour in the psychoses. Finally, I think there is a great deal yet to be done in the study of biogenetics and sound research in child development, although this is still in its early phases. We need to know a great deal about the development of normality in adolescence and adults, and, in various conditions, the adaptations derived from ego functions, particularly in their coping devices.

I have covered the future of psychiatry, as defined both from a medical and scientific point of view, with very broad strokes of the brush. It would be impossible for any one department or institute to cover the entire ground. We are certainly greatly dependent upon the component sciences which make up the whole field of psychiatry. The real problem is to identify these aspects of the various sciences, which contributions or, indeed, which individuals within these sciences we would support as potentially valuable for psychiatry in the near future. It may be that we are entirely dependent upon chance opportunities of getting specific representatives of scientific disciplines to work in a psychiatric department or institute. Many of these people do not feel comfortable working with human behavioural problems, and very frequently state that they like to be with their own kind. This is a contributing factor to the neglect of many important frames of reference for the development of psychiatry. Nevertheless, if we were to establish frequent multidisciplinary discussion groups, or bring representatives of these sciences into the departments for discussions, seminars and conferences, we might maintain at least a superficial grasp of the entire field.

In my opinion, we have to recognise restrictions in what we are capable of doing with our limited space, our limited funds and with those investigators whom we can attract. It may be that some of these overlap within our departments. If there are duplications, then they should be allocated to one place or another. If they do not replicate, but show some indication of variance in approach, I see no reason why the work cannot be independently prosecuted. I do not think that special functions in the vast field of psychiatry can be allocated *a priori*, nor can final decisions be made as to where certain work is carried out.

In delineating the boundaries of modern psychiatry, it is well to remember that the psychiatrist functions solely in the realm of behavioural dysfunction. He is not an expert in dealing with poverty, overpopulation, urban renewal, automation or war. However, he should be capable of dealing expertly with the behavioural difficulties that *might arise* in people who suffer from deprivation, crowding, slums, unemployment or massive stress. Though he may be tempted to overstep the boundaries of his expertise, the psychiatrist lacks the power to implement social action outside the mental health field.

This does not mean that we are sure that what we teach is immutable. What we think we know and teach is for the most part a body of knowledge that gives us only the illusion of certainty. We need to create and innovate, to check continually and evaluate. Thus, it is a sad mistake to separate clinical from research programmes: neither can exist alone.

Questions and answers

1. You refer to a number of professional groups including clinical psychologists and social workers, as 'enemies' of psychiatry. Do you see any prospects for amicable collaboration?

After World War II, we trained and utilised social workers as junior psychiatrists, entrusting them with non-psychotic cases, renaming them psychosocial therapists, and increasing their salaries. But soon clinical psychologists wanted similar treatment, admitting that their PhD degrees were not evidence of interest in research. Their training in the universities was insufficient and they were given fellowships in hospital departments of psychiatry. It was not long before they outnumbered psychiatrists and demanded private offices. They wanted to work on wards, receive equal governmental reimbursement and permission to prescribe medication. They raised large sums of money and fought for equality. Now nurses are following the example of clinical psychologists, and encounter groups with a high level of morbidity are fighting for equality. The outcome cannot be predicted at this time. Actually, all of the mental health professions now are more political than scientific.

2. Though you refer to the need for a general systems theory, you also speak of such global theories as 'escape hatches'. How do you reconcile these statements?

The umbrella of a general theory only encompasses other less global and smaller theories, each one of which may contribute to hypotheses which require well-designed, special operational research.

3. In the light of your personal experience with Freud and your long association with psychoanalysis, how do you now regard the status of the subject?

There is no question that some aspects of psychoanalytical theory are extremely fruitful and would be valuable if they were subjected to operational research. I can think of no more important theoretical formulation applicable to clinical psychiatry than the theory of ego functions, which can be made operational, since ego functions expressed in behaviour are the final common pathways of a wide variety of internal processes. They must, however, be related to situations or environmental conditions and studied from a transactional point of view. Thus, 'insight' is a form of behaviourism. First there is a delineation of action followed by changes in thinking and feeling. Indeed, psychoanalytical theory, when not totally ingested, is helpful in clinical understanding and it is important in understanding the therapist's self and some aspects of a specific patient. But theory devoid of empirical research and understanding has led to superordinate control by an authoritative establishment far removed from science.

Select bibliography

Grinker, R. R., Sr & Stone, T. (1928). Acute toxic encephalitis in childhood. *Archives of Neurology and Psychiatry*, 20, 244–74.

Select bibliography

Grinker, R. R., Sr (1945). *Men Under Stress*. Philadelphia: Blakeston. Paperback (1979), New York: Orrington Press.

Grinker, R. R., Sr & Bucy, P. C. (1949). *Neurology* (4th edition). Oxford: Blackwell Scientific Publications.

Grinker, R. R., Sr (1953). *Mid-century Psychiatry*. Springfield, Illinois: C. C. Thomas.

Grinker, R. R., Sr (1953). *Psychosomatic Research*. New York: W. W. Norton.

Grinker, R. R., Sr (1956). *Towards a Unified Theory of Human Behavior*. New York: Basic Books.

Grinker, R. R., Sr (1962). Mentally healthy young males (Homoclites). *Archives of General Psychiatry*, 6, 405.

Grinker, R. R., Sr (1968). *The Borderline Syndrome*. New York: Basic Books.

Grinker, R. R., Sr (1969). An essay on schizophrenia and science. *Archives of General Psychiatry*, 20, 1–5.

Grinker, R. R., Sr (1969). Psychiatry and our dangerous world. In *Psychiatric Research in our Changing World*, ed. G. F. D. Heseltine, pp. 13–20. Amsterdam: Excerpta Medica Foundation.

Grinker, R. R., Sr (1975). *Psychiatry in Broad Perspective*. New York: Behavior Publications.

Grinker, R. R., Sr (1977). *The Borderline Patient*. New York: Arnoson.

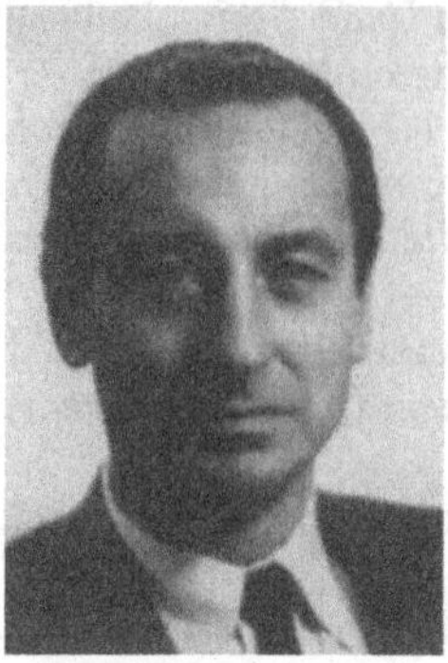

4 · HEINZ HAFNER

Personal background and professional experience

I come from a family that has previously had nothing to do with psychiatry. Since 1540 my ancestors have run a small brewery in Bavaria. Intending at first to study chemistry, I hoped that one day I would be able to make some contribution to knowledge. The war of 1939–45 destroyed these plans and, having been discharged prematurely from military service because of ill-health, I decided in 1944 to study medicine, the only subject permitted in that year. Since medicine did not occupy my time fully, I began to study psychology in 1946 and I took a degree in philosophy at Munich University in 1951.

The decision to start a postgraduate training in psychiatry was based primarily on the wish to commit myself to a branch of medicine that had been seriously damaged by the Third Reich. However, my original goal was not easy to achieve.

After World War II there were few outstanding psychiatrists left in Germany. Both Luxenburger, who before 1933 had carried out epidemiological twin studies at the Kaiser Wilhelm Institute of Psychiatry, and Stertz, who succeeded Bumke in the Chair of Neuropsychiatry at Munich Medical School, advised me to work with Ernst Kretschmer in Tübingen, where I received a very thorough training in psychopathology and psychotherapy. However, I could not adhere to Kretschmer's constitutional theory for long and I already knew Kurt Schneider well and had attended his seminars regularly in Munich.

My own research work at first took three directions: (1) studies in clinical neurology; (2) experimental investigations on the psychology and psychopathology of various forms of cerebral dysfunction; and (3) an interest in existential analysis and in a theory of psychotherapeutic action, both deriving from my philosophical background.

As a consequence of the growing accessibility of the international scientific scene, my judgement of priorities in research was considerably changed. For practical reasons I gradually gave up my interest in neurological subjects and, under the influence especially of British and Scandinavian authors (for example M. Shepherd, J. K. Wing and E. Strömgren), I turned to epidemiological psychiatry in view of its great importance for practice, planning and methods of research in psychiatry. We began to replicate foreign studies and then proceeded to investigate hypotheses of our own with the support, since 1965, of the German Society for the Advancement of Scientific Research ('Special Field of Research: Psychiatric Epidemiology').

Because of the great lack of facilities and staff for research I made efforts to send some staff-members abroad for training, to recruit foreign scientists and to establish a research institute. Since evaluative and health services research were in a bad state and substantial research in psychiatry calls for co-operation with clinical practice, I aimed at a research institute equipped with facilities for the provision of community mental health care. In 1975, 11 years after these plans were first formulated, the Central Institute of Mental Health was opened in Mannheim.

In the difficult period of recovery after the war, it was necessary to endeavour to regain confidence in psychiatry and to carry out fundamental reforms in mental health care. In 1960 we therefore introduced a two-year advanced training in psychiatry for nurses in order to qualify them for taking over new tasks in community psychiatry. Simultaneously, we began to establish complementary services and facilities. Jointly with C. Kulenkampff and W. Picard (Member of Parliament), and with the support of N. Sartorius, J. K. Wing, and D. Bennett, we succeeded in 1968 in bringing the situation of mental health care to the attention of the Federal Parliament. This led to the appointment in 1970 of an expert commission, with which I was closely involved, charged with preparing a report on the state of psychiatry in the Federal Republic of Germany. The proposals of this report helped psychiatry to overcome the difficult period between 1971 and 1976 and ensured its further support. I was then appointed to the Scientific Council, an advisory organ of the Federal Government and the governments of the 10 Länder and West Berlin which carry responsibility for research and training in the universities of Germany. Unfortunately, the growth of bureaucracy and the dwindling financial resources are turning this interesting post into a burden which an active scientist can bear for only a limited time and at a considerable sacrifice.

Current status of psychiatry

Introduction

When asked to give an impression of the current status of one's own field of work, it is difficult to avoid being one-sided. This limitation justifies my focusing on the aspect of psychiatry which I am competent to judge in its historical context, namely the development of the discipline in the German-speaking world. The fact that even today an appropriate criterion of choice can be linguistic has to do with the situation of the subject itself. On the one hand, the scientific foundations of psychiatry and the number of diagnostic and therapeutic techniques that are independent of cultural factors are still limited. On the other hand, the organisation of mental health care and the substance of psychiatric work are more dependent on their cultural and economic framework than is the case with the majority of medical disciplines.

Retrospect

There were many factors common to the development of psychiatry as a separate discipline during the nineteenth century. The Scottish open-door-system, the English non-restraint movement and the ideas of moral treatment spread over the entire European continent and also reached the United States (Meyer, 1863; Jetter, 1971, 1977). The basic works of French and British psychiatrists (for example, Esquirol, 1838; Conolly, 1860) appeared in German soon after they were first published.

The liberal and humanitarian spirit which dominated psychiatry in the train of the bourgeois revolutions led to stagnation in the second half of the nineteenth century. A growing life expectation and the social changes attendant on an industrial society increased the need for psychiatric beds. To a larger degree, however, the teachings of the psychiatrists themselves contributed to a greatly prolonged duration of hospital stay and, as a consequence, to an institutional overcrowding and the development of a passive attitude on the part of formerly active mental hospitals (Brown, 1960). The ideas and achievements of moral treatment and of the social engagement of psychiatric pioneers like Tuke, Esquirol and Conolly mostly fell into oblivion.

The beginnings of 'academic psychiatry'

An academic element was present in the development of German psychiatry from its inception. In 1811 Heinroth was appointed to the first German-speaking chair of 'mental therapy' at the Leipzig Medical School. In 1828 this was renamed the chair of 'psychiatry', a designation introduced by Heinroth himself, who in 1818 published his two-volume German textbook on the disturbances of emotional life. This work is characterised by a strong engagement with moral education. It contains a scheme of 48 psychiatric diagnoses, which was influenced by his teacher Pinel and was based on the theoretical system of human faculties.

Since the need for a communicable classification was strong, while the knowledge of aetiology was poor, academic ambitions concentrated on the development of numerous further classification systems, all of them 'gathered up artificially' (Leubuscher, 1848). Although it was soon recognised that these attempts were useless, they continued to cast their shadows until recently (Stengel, 1958). The early steps towards overcoming such a Babylonian confusion of tongues first went in two directions: (a) the attempt to adopt a restricted somatic nosology and to abandon disease concepts which could not be explained physically, and (b) the attempt to avoid all nosology in favour of comprehensive systems for explaining human behaviour; these systems were expected to provide a basis for localisation along complex dimensions, a form of localisation which can hardly be rendered precise by empirical means, as may be illustrated by the contributions of psychoanalysis.

Neuropsychiatric orientation in German-speaking psychiatry

Animated by the successes and possibilities of scientific medicine and influence by an affiliation to the faculty of medicine, the somatic–nosological orientation became dominant in German-speaking psychiatry. Griesinger, mainly known by the one-sided interpretation of his remark that 'mental diseases are diseases of the brain', was the most influential adherent of this orientation. When he was appointed to the new chair of psychiatry at the University of Berlin, he demanded the establishment of a department of mental disorders. Following this model, all German chairs of this discipline combined psychiatry and neurology until after the Second

World War (the last three major chairs in the Federal Republic – Bonn, Cologne and Erlangen – were split between 1978 and 1981). In many south and east European, Asiatic, African and South American countries this tradition is still preserved.

In 1845, at the age of 28, Griesinger published the first edition of his textbook, anticipating that the segregation of mental hospitals from general hospitals would bring severe disadvantages. He envisaged town asylums – nowadays we would call them psychiatric units in general hospitals – which could provide early treatment for acutely ill patients in co-operation with the other medical disciplines and give aftercare to discharged patients. Even more, he looked forward to the development of psychiatry as a science whose 'mental state' would be maintained in the lap of general medicine and in the face of criticism, '... so that sophisticated bombast, with which at present only in psychiatry something can be done, will soon, here too, give way to sober, clear medical observation'.

Unfortunately, Griesinger's warnings were not able to prevent the progressive isolation of mental state hospitals and its unfavourable consequences. Until the First World War chairs of psychiatry and neurology had been established in nearly all German-speaking universities. The successes achieved in the fields of neuropsychiatry and brain research contributed to the growing reputation of psychiatry within the medical schools and attracted young physicians to take up research and clinical work.

The development of outpatient care

Postgraduate psychiatric training was regulated in the same way as the other medical disciplines. In many countries this enabled the neurologists to engage in private practice, like specialists in internal medicine and surgery. A network of outpatient care rapidly developed, and in those countries with a social security system granting free medical care these outpatient mental health services were provided for everybody and became an integrated part of the mental health care system.

It was probably the early development of a network of easily accessible outpatient services which contributed to the fact that in the Central European countries the proportion of psychiatric beds remained comparably low up to and even after the Second World War. The maximum bed ratio reached between 1950 and 1960 in the Federal Republic of Germany was 1.7/1,000, compared with 4.5/1,000 in the United States, 3.6/1,000 in the United Kingdom, and 5.7/1,000 in Sweden (May, 1976).

Current status of psychiatry

In the majority of Continental countries, except for Swiss psychiatry under the influence of E. Bleuler, the neuropsychiatric medical orientation propagated by the universities determined the nature of outpatient care up to the present day. Its advantages were the relative immunity from ideological thinking and an aversion from assuming any functions which lay beyond its own competence. An essential disadvantage, however, lay in the fact that neuropsychiatrists were insufficiently trained for the treatment of the majority of their patients, particularly those suffering from neuroses. This lack of training in psychotherapy is the decisive reason why general psychiatry has lost important ground to psychoanalysis and psychology.

The neglect of mental hospitals

The general neglect of the mental hospitals until after the Second World War was also a feature of German-speaking psychiatry. In part at least, it can be ascribed to the isolation of mental hospital psychiatry from the rest of medicine, as predicted by Griesinger, and to the related stagnation of research, treatment and general care.

It may be mentioned that both the neuropsychiatrically oriented psychiatrists in Europe and their analytically inclined colleagues in North America exhibited all too little concern for the mental hospitals in the pre-war years. However, this general trend does not account for the darkest chapter in the history of German psychiatry: the compulsory sterilisation and euthanasia of the mentally ill during the Nazi era. Even though it had been announced in early psychiatric publications (Binding & Hoche, 1920), this intrusion of inhumanity is explicable only in the context of the Nazi ideology of extermination (Mitscherlich & Mielke, 1962; Ehrhardt, 1965). The post-war development of psychiatry in the states succeeding the Third Reich in West and East Germany and in Austria was profoundly influenced by this extraordinary period. Scientific links with foreign countries were interrupted for about one decade. The number of senior psychiatrists who had not corrupted themselves politically was small, and it took more than 20 years of regeneration before scientific work in psychiatry recommenced on any scale.

The classification of mental disorders

For a very long time the lack of a commonly accepted nomenclature, based on sufficiently precise and validated diagnostic constructs, had been the main obstacle to the process of psychiatric research. In 1958, Stengel stated in a WHO report that, in addition to the International Classification of Diseases (ICD), at that time accepted by very few countries, 38 national or individual schemes for diagnosing mental disturbances were in use. According to an estimate by Beck and his colleagues (Beck, 1962; Beck, Ward, Mendelson,. Mock & Erbough, 1962), deficient classificatory schemata played a large part in accounting for the unreliability of many psychiatric diagnoses, a phenomenon which discredited the discipline in the eyes of many observers. Opponents of any labelling system (for example Szasz, 1960; Scheff, 1966), it may be observed, still neglect the necessary distinction between the singularity of the individual and the necessity of an inter-individual comparability of symptoms and the regular course of a disease which serve as a basis for the precise assignment of a 'case' to a diagnostic category, with all the consequences for communication, prognosis and treatment.

As a result of the initiatives taken by the Mental Health Division of the WHO and under the influence of British, Scandinavian and some American workers (for example the St Louis School), the interest in an empirical and taxonomic system of diagnoses has nonetheless greatly increased in recent years. In retrospect the German predecessors of this development – Kraepelin, Jaspers and Kurt Schneider – may now be seen to have exerted a pronounced influence on the psychiatry of our day. In the fourth edition of his textbook (1893), Kraepelin had laid the foundation for the present system of diagnosing mental disturbances. Realising that the small number of diseases with an established aetiology did not permit a comprehensive nosological classification, he tried to introduce 'preliminary disease units' by describing symptoms, syndromes and courses in the tradition of Thomas Sydenham. On the basis of his clinical experience, Kraepelin continually reviewed his disease concepts and their systematic assignment and altered them several times. An empirical system of this kind, composed of heterogeneous categories, cannot meet the requirements for a scientific classification; however, it is of great empirical value for psychiatry (Shepherd, 1976). Kraepelin's hopes of obtaining a 'natural classification' of mental disorders by means of a profound knowledge of aetiology, symptomatology and pathological anatomy was not to be realised. The fact that different somatic diseases may produce the same psychiatric disturbances and that one and the same disease may take a different course discouraged him to such an extent that at the end of his life he cast doubt on the value of his entire life's work.

Nevertheless, his unprejudiced empirical approach to a taxonomic system of psychiatric disorders survived him, as did some of his main disease constructs. They do not depend on a comprehensive theory of human behaviour and are not restricted to a somatic nosology. In consequence, Kraepelin made the first successful attempt to develop an empirically based diagnostic system which can be applied to all psychiatric disorders.

The descriptive psychopathology of the 'Heidelberg School'

Kraepelin's work found its complement in Karl Jaspers' *Allgemeine Psychopathologie* (General Psychopathology) (1913). The 'Heidelberg School' (including H. Gruhle, W. Mayer-Gross, K. Schneider) originated with Jaspers and adopted his taxonomic system, which was founded on the separation of psychological understanding and causal explanation, on the distinction between process and development, and between somatogenic and psychogenic aetiological disturbances. The logic of empirical research played no role in this schema. Knowledge was based entirely on 'evidence'.

However, a surprising degree of precision was reached in the description and assignment of psychopathological phenomena. For example, the cultural validity of the first rank symptoms of nuclear schizophrenia, compiled by Kurt Schneider solely from clinical observation, were supported by high cross-national rates of agreement (WHO, 1973).

Mobilisation of potential for research

Since the commencement of its Programme on Standardisation, Classification and Statistics in 1966, the World Health Organisation has been making successful efforts to improve the definitions and taxonomy of psychiatric diagnoses in relation to the ICD (Shepherd, Brooke, Cooper & Lin, 1968; Sartorius, Brooke & Lin, 1970). At present the eighth and the ninth revisions of the ICD are being used in almost all countries except the United States, which still adheres to a Monroe Doctrine of mental health, and a few francophonic countries. As a consequence, the prerequisites for an international use of existing research potential are much improved.

Precisely defined constructs of diagnoses have also made it possible to develop objective and reliable methods for the assessment of diagnoses or syndromes and for case identification. For the first time the scientific demands for reproducible and replicable findings can be satisfied in many fields of psychiatry. An essential basis for current psychiatric research has come from this development.

Biological psychiatry

In German-speaking areas biological psychiatry has been able to continue in the formerly renôwned neuropsychiatric tradition; it has succeeded in improving the tarnished reputation of the discipline in the medical world. There is an increasing confidence in the prospects of establishing specific biochemical or neurophysiological correlates of mental disorder, but until now this has only been supported to a small extent. Meanwhile, there have been important achievements in the understanding of the neurochemical actions of psychotropic drugs. These alone already guarantee fruitful advances in this sphere of research.

It has still to be determined, however, which biological disturbances are caused by particular diseases, which are mainly provoked by the reaction of the person affected and which are due to non-specific factors. Since the causal intermediate links between psychiatric disturbances and biological changes are largely unknown, a broad spectrum of hypotheses has to be pursued. The variety of biological findings considered to be relevant might perhaps be reduced by the identification of those changes occurring in healthy individuals as a result of comparable states of anxiety, stress, activity or inactivity.

The problem posed by the logical assignment of the multiple psychogenic and somatogenic phenomena discussed by Kraepelin and the increasing knowledge of the importance of genetic, neurophysiological, neurobiochemical, social and psychological factors for the development, onset and prognosis of some psychiatric disorders, introduce a high level of complexity into psychiatric research and practice. Because of its involvement with various levels of phenomena and with a wide variety of methodologies, psychiatry has to cope with increasing difficulties in the processing and circulation of information.

The complexity of diagnostic information can be met by introducing dimensional instead of categorical diagnostic constructs. For many research purposes this approach has to be adopted because it allows assessment on various levels and improves the possibilities of statistical processing. In practice, however, the clumsiness and often also the lack of obvious clinical relevance of some constructs, especially of mathematically derived constructs, raise difficulties. Nevertheless, dimensional diagnoses must be employed if a disease comprises various and differing dimensions of disorders. In mental retardation, for instance, at the lower levels of intelligence the dimensions of IQ, the development of language, social competence and a number of sensory defects diverge significantly (Cooper, Liepmann, Marker & Schieber, 1979). In order to obtain a diagnosis which is related to the needs, the application of a 'handicaps schedule' has been proposed (Bernson, 1980; Wing, 1980). This model can probably also be used for the diagnosis of comparable disturbances in other conditions, such as disability after schizophrenia.

'Multi-axial' diagnosis can be regarded as a compromise, since it fulfils the need to record important information on various levels while maintaining categorical diagnostic concepts. In child and adolescent psychiatry, it has been successfully tested in a WHO study (Rutter, Shaffer & Sturge, 1975) and has since been introduced internationally (Remschmidt, Schmidt & Klicpera, 1977).

Problems of the 'minor' mental disorders

Despite the progress made in the taxonomy and validation of psychiatric diagnoses, diagnostic systems and constructs are still unsatisfactory in the field of the so-called 'minor' mental disorders (neuroses, personality disorders, etc.). The indications for available forms of treatment, such as anxiolytic drugs, behaviour therapy or psychoanalysis, are rarely determined by diagnoses, but by 'target symptoms' or by behavioural concepts. Both psychoanalysis and the German 'understanding psychopathology', as represented by such writers as Kretschmer and Tellenbach, have contributed interesting models for the explanation of the regularity of development and course of these disorders. However, most of these models have not been verified by empirical methods; nor have they led to an effective therapeutic strategy. It can be expected that the explanatory models of behaviour therapy will have better chances of experimental verification: different forms of learned maladaptive behaviour may be eliminated or corrected by appropriate learning processes. The progress which has been achieved in, for instance, the cognitive therapy of chronic depressions (Seligman, 1975; Beck, Rush, Shaw & Emery, 1979) and the treatment of anxiety and obsessional neuroses leads to the assumption that these developments have still to be explored. There is some chance that, with the knowledge gained, dimensions or new constructs will be found which might be of use for the construction of diagnoses because of their heuristic and predictive value. Such a development may lead to an elaboration or a new taxonomy of the minor mental disorders which constitute so large a burden of morbidity as to underline the importance of the search for a broader, more rational basis of diagnosis and treatment.

Psychiatry and psychoanalysis

Psychoanalysis developed in Germany and Austria at a time when academic psychiatry was still adhering to its neuropsychiatric orientation. This is indisputably one of the reasons why psychoanalysis was kept apart from the German-speaking universities, except for Zurich (E. Bleuler), and, as a consequence, kept apart from scientific discussions for more than half a century. At the same time the far-reaching claims of Freud's explanatory model and the special demands of psychoanalytical training also constituted an obstacle to a broad empirical examination of psychoanalytical propositions. Nonetheless, an enormous revival of psychoanalysis took place in Central Europe from the 1960s, an event which can be understood partially as an expression of the need to make amends for its previous exclusion. In Switzerland psychoanalytical training became an indispensable component of postgraduate training in psychiatry. In the Federal Republic an extensive reform of medical training introduced the new compulsory subject of 'psychotherapy and psychosomatic medicine'. Meanwhile, chairs of psychotherapy have been established at all 25 medical schools. The majority of these chairs are held by psychoanalysts.

As a consequence of these developments medical students are no longer trained by general psychiatrists in the diagnosis and the treatment of psycho-reactive disorders. Instead, psychoanalysts soon make them familiar with psychodynamic concepts and interpretations of minor mental and the so-called psychosomatic disorders. In 1972, at a time of economic prosperity, social insurance began to include psychoanalytical group or individual treatment among its benefits, and since then it has been paying relatively high rates to psychotherapists and psychoanalysts. In 1980 a first step in the same direction was made towards the acceptance of behaviour therapy by qualified clincial psychologists. It seems likely, however, that the economic recession will slow down a further extension of such paid benefits.

This development raises a major question in the field of health policy: can the community be burdened with the treatment of individuals who are on the borderline between health and disease, at a cost of large sums expended on a relatively small number of persons, when the improvement of the situation of many chronic patients must be postponed because the costs cannot be covered? A further problem arises from the growing interest of young psychiatric residents in analytical training, since for the moment it guarantees a good income from social insurance and less competition in practice. In addition, psychoanalytical training seems to attract those physicians who feel a dislike for the precise and economical thinking associated with the natural sciences. It seems to promote associative thought strategies and leads to the neglect of causal–discursive modes of thinking (Leuzinger, 1980). In the future it will be decisive for the new professors of psychotherapy to question their traditional concepts and commit themselves increasingly to empirical research, especially in the field of conceptualisation and the indications for and evaluation of psychotherapeutic methods.

Future prospects of psychiatry

The questions that I have raised must be seen in the context of an issue which is vital for the future of psychiatry. What is to be the psychiatrist's sphere of professional competence in the fields of mental health care, training and research? On the somatic side, psychiatry has already lost a large segment of its functions to neurology and neurosurgery. Like internal medicine, it has handed over to neighbouring disciplines the responsibility for those diseases, for example general paresis and brain tumours, whose aetiology is known and which can be treated with new techniques. It retains the large number of poorly understood mental disorders which can be treated without much technology, and future research will have to concentrate on the core of this spectrum of disorders.

However, the development of research usually follows the process of specialisation. Technological advances and successful research attract gifted scientists and financial support. Underdeveloped technologies, poorly defined models of diseases and unclear therapeutic indications are more likely to deter both individual scientists and research institutions. The advancement of research is therefore mostly supported where progress has been apparent. This difficulty should be met by setting priorities for research promotion.

At the other end of the spectrum general psychiatry is being threatened by the loss of its competence in the field of psychotherapy. In addition to the independent status of psychotherapy at the universities and the claims of psychoanalysts for participation in mental health care, clinical psychologists are demanding that they take over all non-psychoanalytical methods of treatment. The situation is not yet comparable to that obtaining in the United States, where the number of psychologists and social workers far exceeds that of psychiatrists working in community mental health centres. However, since in future the annual numbers of qualifying psychiatrists and psychologists will be about 300 to 400 and 2,000 to 2,200 respectively, similar problems are on the horizon.

Good psychiatry is dependent on psychological methods. These are needed not only for the treatment of reactive disorders but also for the investigation, diagnosis and treatment of endogenous and exogenous disorders. In consequence, the training of psychiatric residents must include instruction in all these methods. Two pre-conditions are indispensable for a successful defence of this requirement in the light of the claims made by the new academic discipline of psychotherapy and by an intensively research-oriented psychology. First, high-quality research must be carried out in the nuclear field of psychiatry in order to improve rational diagnosis, treatment and prevention. Secondly, the broad zone of overlap in research, training and health care must be acknowledged and tackled by means of high-quality interdisciplinary collaboration.

Many of the difficulties are well illustrated by the current situation in state mental hospitals. The frequency of hospital admissions for schizophrenia and affective psychoses is decreasing sharply as a result of the provision of a wider network of outpatient services, the increasing number of physicians and the creation of complementary facilities. In spite of the low figure of 1.7 beds per 1,000 population, the number of beds occupied in mental hospitals has been decreasing by 20 per cent on average; 40 to 50 per cent of the patients are admitted for alcohol-related diseases. Griesinger's predicted consequences of isolation are being confirmed.

A secondary phase of neglect and a lowering of morale in the mental hospital staff can be countered only by means of far-reaching changes of the care system, as was recently recommended by the World Health Organisation (1978). However, these reforms will take time, for the transition to community mental health care is expensive, especially the establishment of psychiatric units in general hospitals and the modernisation of those mental hospitals which are suited to take over special functions or to become an integral part of the community mental health care system. In the United States, as a consequence of the mental health movement and the Community Mental Health Care programme, American psychiatry has had to cope with an extreme enlargement of its domain. This has not occurred in German-speaking countries, where the reputation of the discipline has not suffered a comparable decline (Brody, 1972; Torrey, 1974). In 1975, an expert parliamentary commission submitted its report on the state of mental health care in the Federal Republic of Germany. Based on a broad consensus of psychiatric opinion, this report recommended a sensible reform of mental health care, clearly influenced by the recommendations of WHO and by the experience of the United Kingdom. The ideas laid down in the expert's report have also had some effect on the plans being pursued in Austria, Switzerland and East Germany.

At present, greater problems arise from a somewhat irrational campaign conducted by the mass media, mainly by laymen. This is directed against all somatic therapy, but also against 'manipulative' psychological methods of treatment and sometimes even against the very existence of psychiatry. Behind this trend lies not only the old conviction that mental disorders may be assessed adequately by the lay public and healed by encouragement, but also the popularisation of certain theories propagated by social scientists, for instance the theory of symbolic interactionism (Scheff, 1966) and the assumption that family processes are themselves pathogenic (Stierlin, 1975).

These confusing opinions create a feeling of insecurity, especially among the mentally ill who, unlike many physically sick people, are unable to understand the nature of their disorders, where they can obtain competent help and what chances of recovery they have. New efforts, preferably beginning in the school years, should be taken to furnish the population, with information about mental disorders and the provisions for treatment.

Psychiatry is at a critical phase of its history. It is threatened not only by the loss of several of its peripheral spheres of activity but also by assaults on its central tasks in respect of research and treatment. Can psychiatry compensate for the erosion of its territory by attempting to expand? The example of the United States provides a clear answer: the boundaries of its competence must not exceed the limits of effective action. Its legitimate domain still remains sufficiently large, covering many subjects and areas of research and practice with which other specialties must occupy themselves. With regard to the broad zones of overlap in research and practice, some competition will be inevitable, perhaps even fruitful. However, the future of psychiatry lies in the quality of its scientific and therapeutic work, which meanwhile must be essentially interdisciplinary. In the dialogue with representatives of neighbouring disciplines, critical discussion of one-sided or over-generalised theories or results will assume increasing importance. Such discussion might contribute a successful way of enlarging the rational ground of psychiatric action and of dissipating the cloud of irrationality which disconcerts both psychiatrists and patients.

HEINZ HAFNER

Questions and answers

1. You refer to 'priorities for research promotion'. What 'priorities' would you recommend?

My priorities in the field of mental health research are chosen partly to serve as a counterweight to the technological outlook to which I have referred but mainly to draw attention to the important public health aspects in the field of psychiatric research. This is why some important topics in current research – for instance, the biochemistry of neurotransmitters in connection with the onset, course and treatment of the functional psychoses – will not be mentioned.

One has to consider differences in priorities between developing countries and industrialised nations. These are due to differences in the urgency of the problems and to variations in resources of manpower, research equipment and technology. Thus, for international research a certain degree of division of labour seems to be necessary if we are to avoid status-bound, low-quality research and an unfavourable concentration on a few opportune research questions. This should not constitute a hindrance to the replication of investigations as an instrument for scientific verification or falsification. A minimum of co-ordination is also necessary to obtain a response to research results from those bodies who are mainly interested, that is governments, health authorities and the medical profession itself; in this way we can come to know whether the most essential mental health problems have been tackled. The World Health Organisation's Division of Mental Health has been making successful efforts in this direction.

In more detail, I would categorise my priorities as follows:

(a) *Epidemiology and social psychiatry*

(i) *Mental health and environment.* Here, I would stress the influence of the cultural and social background on the mental health of the individual and the population, especially the impact of family bonds (Henderson, 1980) and the changes in family and sociocultural structures and other systems regulating human behaviour (for example, education) compared with the impact of particular aspects of social anomie. The relevance and predictability of the social environment for the health of individuals or certain categories of individuals or diseases also call for study. As an extreme case I would mention that the success of token economy programmes in chronic schizophrenics could be due to the fact that they make an arbitrary and complex environment, i.e. the mental hospital, more predictable for socially disabled patients (Cohen, 1981).

(ii) *The transmission of behaviour patterns affecting health*. In this field I would single out the investigation of the communicability and spread of the mechanisms and the manner of disseminating behaviour which may affect mental health, for example parasuicidal acts (Phillips, 1974; Welz, 1980), drug and alcohol abuse (de Alarcón, 1969; Chambers, 1976) and patterns of chronic depressive behaviour. The identification of genetic, social, familial and individual factors associated with low or high risk for such behaviour patterns is also important, along with the identification of factors protecting against risk behaviour and relapses of mental disorders.

(iii) *The genetics of mental disorder and health affecting behaviour*. The focus of further research in this field should be more connected with attempts to identify genetic markers or comparable phenomena associated with the genotype rather than with an increasing number of descriptive studies based only on phenotypes.

(iv) *Prevention, therapy and rehabilitation*. For the purposes of intervention evaluation is demanded of several intra- and non-professional and extra-familial techniques for managing life crises, severe neurotic problems and the functional psychoses. The effectiveness of self-help groups comes into this category.

Much more work is needed for a precise and valid assessment of the so-called 'basic impairment' contributing mainly to disability following severe neurotic and functional mental disorders (Jablensky, Schwarz & Tomov, 1980; WHO, 1973). An analysis of the onset and course of impairment and of its dependence of disease-linked and environmental factors should be feasible, followed by the development and evaluation of specific psychological training measures designed to influence or compensate for these impairments and thus to reduce the disability.

(b) *Basic research*

(i) *Psychophysiology* There should be further development of analytic procedures in order to derive better neurophysiological indicators, for example the EEG-parameters of mental functions such as changes in attention. The prevailing objectives are to detect and to explain the psychophysiological correlates of functional mental disorders (Koukkou & Lehmann, 1980; Gasser, Verleger, Möcks, Bächer & Lederer, 1981.

(ii) *Neurochemistry as a basis for treatment with psychoactive drugs*. Current investigations on neurotransmitter metabolism and its functions must be pursued. The topography and pharmacology of receptors within the CNS may lead to the discovery of antipsychotic substances with fewer anti-cholinergic and other side effects, such as tardive dyskinesia (Beckmann & Haas, 1980).

(iii) *The mental health of children and adolescents.* Longitudinal studies on children at risk and/or with perinatal problems are needed to obtain information about the etiology, prognosis and prevention of behaviour disorders, especially of so-called minimal brain damage. Two problem areas have to be tackled: (a) the investigation or control of genetic and environmental factors, such as social background, family and school education; and (b) the development of the age-related standardisation of replicable methods of assessing social, mental, neurological and neurophysiological functioning.

(iv) *Mental health of the elderly.* Work is needed on mental and social functioning and self-satisfaction related to passivity, dependency and depression in old age. In particular, it would be important to establish predictors associated with, and factors responsible for, these aspects of mental health in the elderly.

2. You suggest that the future of psychiatry resides in 'interdisciplinary' work. Precisely what forms of interdisciplinary work do you have in mind?

(a) *University education* In many European countries – for instance, in the Federal Republic of Germany – university education in psychology and the study of medicine as a basis for postgraduate training in psychiatry are completely separate. During their studies psychologists never or rarely see a mentally ill patient and their knowledge of the field of mental health remains theoretical. Medical students, by the same token, receive very little instruction in the psychological methods employed for diagnosis, therapy or research. For such work it is imperative to include both more basic knowledge and more clinical experience to lay the foundations of postgraduate training in the field of mental health, especially in view of the importance of education in interdisciplinary research.

(b) *Interdisciplinary organisation of research training and research in the field of mental health* Each university department of psychiatry should, in my opinion, include a department or at least a unit of clinical and research psychology, because psychodiagnostics and psychological forms of interventions, for example behaviour therapy, as well as psychological research methods are indispensable components of clinical and research education in psychiatry. For the same reason each department of psychotherapy and psychosomatic medicine should be closely linked with the psychiatric department, even if it is attached to a department of internal medicine.

In some places a fruitful culture of inter-disciplinary interests and knowledge has been created by the gathering together under one roof of different departments with an interest in psychiatric research. In a few universities and research institutes psychiatric departments or research units should be sufficiently equipped to be in a position to pursue particular interdisciplinary aspects of psychiatric research, such as neurochemistry, psychophysiology or the behavioural aspects of psychosomatic medicine. In this way it would be possible to bring research workers in the basic sciences directly in touch with clinical problems. They might also be stimulated to co-operate with skilled psychiatrists who had acquired a knowledge of basic research methods during their postgraduate training; this would facilitate mutual understanding. The fields of epidemiology and health services research provide examples demanding indispensable interdisciplinary co-operation involving psychiatrists, psychologists, sociologists and biostatisticians. Other specialists would have to join the nuclear team for the investigation of special fields; for instance, an economist would be required for cost-benefit analyses.

In addition to permanent research facilities, there is a case for the promotion of project teams coming from different institutions, and for medium-term methods of interdisciplinary target research combining the skills of different institutions. As an example I would mention the 'Special Research Units' (*Sonderforschungsbereiche*) in the Federal Republic of Germany, which are composed of interdisciplinary groups of research workers coming from different institutes and co-operating for a period of 10 to 15 years in order to work on a defined research topic.

(c) *Practical work* The interdisciplinary integration of practical psychiatric work demands, above all, a basis of community mental health services. Co-operation with general practitioners and general hospitals should be emphasised here. In the latter case the priority area is the emergency service in which psychiatry should be represented principally for the care of incurably ill patients. Of particular relevance to interdisciplinary co-operation are those illnesses for which behavioural medicine is of special importance.

3. What forms of empirical research do you recommend for the new German Professors of Psychotherapy?

(a) *Diagnosis and classification* They should be involved in the continuation of international efforts to improve the definition and validation of sufficiently discriminating and consistent constructs of diagnoses in the field of the so-called minor mental disorders as a prerequisite for a better taxonomy of the neuroses and personality disorders.

(b) *Basic research on abnormal behaviour* They should participate in the analysis of those behavioural, motivational or cognitive strategies which may underlie specific clusters of neurotic symptoms or deviant behaviour. For example, there could be an operationalisation of selected and suitable psychoanalytical assumptions – like the model of regression progressing with increasing anxiety – in order to arrive at the verification or falsification of clearly defined hypotheses.

(c) *Research in therapeutic techniques and their evaluation* Investigations on specific or non-specific indications of psychological or psychotherapeutic interventions in connection with evaluative approaches are needed to establish which methods are efficient, inefficient or harmful in particular disorders, behaviour patterns or diseases.

(d) *The role of non-professional help potentials* An assessment of psychotherapeutic intervention in relation to assistance provided by the family and lay helpers is long overdue.

(e) *Psychophysiology and psychosomatics* Psychotherapists should concern themselves with paradigms or models for psychophysiological processes and reactions in relation to risk behaviour, stress, and the processes underlying the development of certain 'psychosomatic' diseases or disease-like functional disorders. They should attempt to close the gap between psychophysiological research and health problems. An increase in their contributions to behavioural medicine would be useful, for example by an examination of forms of individual or group behaviour as risk factors for the onset and adverse outcome of such physical illnesses as diabetes or cardiovascular diseases, and by studies of the influence of behavioural factors on the success of psychotherapeutic, surgical and drug treatments. Finally, psychotherapists should participate more in the investigation of direct associations between emotional processes and learning processes as well as behaviour patterns on the one hand, and physiological parameters or bodily functions, such as digestion, cardiac output and blood pressure, on the other hand.

References

Alarcón, R. de (1969). The spread of heroin in a community. *Bulletin on Narcotics*, **21**, 17–22.

Beck, A. T. (1962). Reliability of psychiatric diagnoses: 1. A critique of systematic studies. *American Journal of Psychiatry*, **119**, 210–16.

Beck, A. T., Ward, C. H., Mendelson, M., Mock, J. E. & Erbough, J. K. (1962). Reliability of psychiatric diagnoses: 2. A study of consistency of clinical judgements and ratings. *American Journal of Psychiatry*, **119**, 351–7.

Beck, A. T., Rush, A. J., Shaw, B. F. & Emery, G. (1979). *Cognitive Therapy of Depression*. New York: Guilford.

Beckmann, H. & Haas, St. (1980). High dose diazepam in schizophrenia. *Psychopharmacology*, **71**, 79–82.

Bericht über die Lage der Psychiatrie in der Bundesrepublik Deutschland – Zur Psychiatrischen und psychotherapeutisch/psychosomatischen Versorgung der Bevölkerung (1975). Bonn, Deutscher Bundestag, Drs. 7/4200, 7/4201.

Bernson, A. H. (1980). The children's Handicaps, Behaviour and Skills (HBS) Schedule. A report on its reliability under Danish conditions. In *Epidemiological Research as Basis for the Organization of Extramural Psychiatry*, ed. E. Strömgren, A. Dupont & J. A. Nielson, pp. 133–9. Copenhagen: Munksgaard.

Binding, K. & Hoche, A. (1920). *Die Freigabe der Vernichtung lebensunwerten Lebens*. Leipzig: F. Meiner.

Brody, E. B. (1972). Models in psychiatric education. *Journal of Nervous and Mental Disease*, **154**, 153–6.

Brown, G. W. (1960). Length of hospital stay and schizophrenia. A review of statistical studies. *Acta Psychiatrica et Neurologica Scandinavica*, **35**, 414–30.

Chambers, C. D. & Hunt, L. G. (1976). *The Heroin Epidemics*. New York: Spectrum Publications.

Cohen, R. (1981). Indikation und Kontraindikation von Token Economy Verfahren bei chronisch Schizophrenen. In *Psychotherapie in der Psychiatrie*, ed. H. Helmchen, M. Linden & U. Rüger. Heidelberg, Berlin & New York: Springer Verlag.

Conolly, J. (1860). *Die Behandlung der Irren ohne mechanischen Zwang*. (English translation (1856) *Treatment of the insane without mechanical restraints*. Lahr: Schauenburg.

Cooper, B., Liepmann, M. C., Marker, K. R. & Schieber, P. M. (1979). Definition of severe mental retardation in school-age children: findings of an epidemiological study. *Social Psychiatry*, **14**, 197–205.

Ehrhardt, H. (1965). *Euthanasie und Vernichtung 'lebensunwerten' Lebens*. Stuttgart: Enke Verlag.

Esquirol, J. E. D. (1838). *Des Maladies Mentales*. J. B. Baillière, Libraire de l'Académie Royale de Médecine, vol. 2, p. 723. Paris.

Gasser, Th., Verleger, R., Möcks, J., Bächer, P. & Lederer, W. M. (1981). The EEG patterns of mildly retarded children: clinical and quantitative

findings. In *Assessing the Handicaps and Needs of Mentally Retarded Children*, ed. B. Cooper, pp. 79–89. London: Academic Press.
Griesinger, W. (1845). *Die Pathologie und Therapie der psychischen Krankheiten*. Stuttgart: Krabbe Verlag.
Heinroth, J. C. A. (1818). *Lehrbuch der Störungen des Seelenlebens oder der Seelenstörungen und ihrer Behandlung*. Ed. I u. II. Leipzig: Vogel Verlag.
Henderson, S. (1980). A development in social psychiatry. The systematic of social bonds. *The Journal of Nervous and Mental Disease*, **168**, 63–9.
Jablensky, A., Schwarz, R. & Tomov, T. (1980). WHO collaborative study on impairments and disabilities associated with schizophrenic disorders. A preliminary communication: objectives and methods. In *Epidemiological Research as Basis for the Organization of Extramural Psychiatry*, ed. E. Strömgren, A. Dupont & J. A. Nielson *Acta Psychiatrica Scandinavica*, Supplement 285, vol. 62, pp. 152–63. Copenhagen: Munksgaard.
Jaspers, K. (1965). *Allgemeine Psychopathologie* (8. Auflage). Berlin, Heidelberg & New York: Springer Verlag.
Jetter, D. (1971). *Zur Typologie des Irrenhauses in Frankreich und Deutschland (1780–1840)*. Wiesbaden: Steiner Verlag.
Jetter, D. (1977). *Grundzüge der Krankenhausgeschichte (1800–1900)*. Darmstadt: Wissenschaftliche Buchgesellschaft.
Koukkou, M. & Lehmann, D. (1980). Brain functional states: determinants, constraints and implications. In *Functional States of the Brain: their Determinants*, ed. M. Koukkou, D. Lehmann & J. Angst, pp. 13–22, Amsterdam, New York & Oxford: Elsevier.
Kraepelin, E. (1893). *Psychiatrie. Ein kurzes Lehrbuch für Studirende und Aerzte* (4th edition). Leipzig: Ambr. Abel.
Leubuscher, R. (1848). Die Irrenverhältnisse Berlin's. *Die Medicinische Reform*, **17**, 119–20; **18**, 127–9; **20**, 141–3.
Leuzinger, A. (1980). Kognitive Prozesse bei der Indikationsstellung zur Psychotherapie. Vortrag auf dem Symposion *Indikation zur Psychotherapie*, 29–31. 10. 1980, Werner Reimers Stiftung, Bad Homburg.
May, A. R. (1976). *Mental Health Services in Europe*. A review of data collected in response to a WHO questionnaire. Geneva: World Health Organisation.
Meyer, L. (1863). Das non-restraint und die deutsche Psychiatrie. *Allgemeine Zeitschrift für Psychiatrie*, **20**, 542–81.
Mitscherlich, A. & Mielke, I. (ed.) (1962). *Medizin ohne Menschlichkeit. Dokumente des Nürnberger Arzteprozesses*. Frankfurt: Fischer Verlag.
Phillips, D. P. (1974). The influence of suggestion on suicide: Substantive and theoretical implications of the 'Werther effect'. *American Sociological Review*, **39**, 340–54.
Remschmidt, H., Schmidt, M. & Klicpera, C. (ed.) (1977). *Multiaxiales Klassifikationsschema für psychiatrische Erkrankungen im Kindes- und Jugendalter nach Rutter, Shaffer und Sturge*. Bern, Stuttgart & Wien: Huber Verlag.
Rutter, M., Shaffer, D. & Sturge, C. (1975). *A Guide to a Multi-Axial Classification Scheme for Psychiatric Disorders in Childhood and Adolescence*. London: Department of Child and Adolescent Psychiatry.

Sartorius, N., Brooke, E. M. & Lin, T. (1970). Reliability of psychiatric assessment in international research. In *Psychiatric Epidemiology*, ed. E. Hare & J. K. Wing pp. 133–47. London: Oxford University Press.

Scheff, Th. J. (1966). *Being Mentally Ill*. Chicago: Aldine.

Seligman, M. E. P. (1975). *Helplessness. On Depression, Development and Death*. San Francisco: W.H. Freeman & Co.

Shepherd, M. (1976). Definition, classification and nomenclature: a clinical overview. In *Schizophrenia Today*, ed. D. Kemali, G. Bartholini & D. Ritcher, pp. 3–12. Oxford: Pergamon Press.

Shepherd, M., Brooke, E. M., Cooper, J. E. & Lin, T. (1968). An experimental approach to psychiatric diagnosis. *Acta Psychiatrica Scandinavica*, Supplement 201.

Stengel, E. (1958). Classification of mental disorders. *Bulletin of the World Health Organisation*, **21**, 601–63.

Stierlin, H. (1975). *Von der Psychoanalyse zur Familientherapie*. Stuttgart: Klett Verlag.

Szasz, T. S. (1960). The myth of mental illness. *American Psychologist*, **15**, 113–18.

Torrey, E. F. (1974). *The Death of Psychiatry*. Radnor, Pa.: Cilton.

Welz, R. (1980). Suicidal areas: cluster analysis profiles of urban environments. In *Epidemiological Research as Basis for the Organization of Extramural Psychiatry*, ed. E. Strömgren, A. Dupont & J. A. Nielson. *Acta Psychiatrica Scandinavica*, Supplement 285, vol. 62, pp. 372–81. Copenhagen: Munksgaard.

Wing, L. (1980). The MRC Handicaps, Behaviour & Skills (HBS) schedule. In *Epidemiological Research as Basis for the Organization of Extramural Psychiatry*, ed. E. Strömgren, A. Dupont & J. A. Neilson, pp. 242–27. Copenhagen: Munksgaard.

World Health Organisation (1973). *The International Pilot Study of Schizophrenia*. Vol. 1. Geneva: World Health Organisation.

World Health Organisation, Regional Office for Europe (1978). *The Future of Mental Hospitals*. Report on a Working Group, Mannheim, 2–5 November 1976. Copenhagen: ICP/MNH 019 II.

Select bibliography

Häfner, H. (1953). Uber Wahrnehmungs- und Bedeutungsstrukturen und ihre Beziehungen zur emotionalen Einstellung. *Zeitschrift für experimentelle und angewandte Psychologie*, **4**, 568–604.

Häfner, H. (1953). Psychopathologie der cerebralorganisch bedingten Zeitsinnesstörungen. *Archiv für Psychiatrie und Zeitschrift Neurologie*, Band **190**, 530–45.

Häfner, H. (1954). Die existentielle Depression. *Archiv für Psychiatrie und Zeitschrift Neurologie*, Band **191**, 351–64.

Häfner, H. (1954). Zur Psychopathologie der halluzinatorischen Schizophrenie. *Archiv für Psychiatrie und Zeitschrift Neurologie*, Band **192**, 241–58.

Häfner, H. (1956). *Schulderleben und Gewissen*. Stuttgart: Klett.

Häfner, H. (1958). Uber sensitive Charakterentwicklung. Mehrdimensionale Diagnostik und Therapie. In *Festschrift zum 70. Geburtstag von Herrn Professor Dr. med. Dr. phil. h.c. Ernst Kretschmer*, pp. 101–10. Stuttgart: Thieme.

Häfner, H. (1963). Prozeß und Entwicklung als Grundbegriffe der Psychopathologie. *Fortschritte der Neurologie, Psychiatrie*, **31**, 393–438.

Baeyer v., W., Häfner, H. & Kisker, K. P. (1964). *Psychiatrie der Verfolgten*. Berlin, Heidelberg & Göttingen: Springer.

Vogel, F., Häfner, H. & Diebold K. (1965). Zur Genetik der progressiven Myoklonusepilepsien (Unverricht-Lundborg). *Humangenetik*, **1**, 437–75.

Diebold, K., Häfner, H., Vogel, F. & Schalt, E. (1968). Die myoklonischen Varianten der familiären amaurotischen Idiotie. *Humangenetik*, **5**, 119–4.

Häfner, H. (1968). Psychological disturbances following prolonged persecution. *Social Psychiatry*, **3**, 79–88.

Häfner, H., Reimann, H. Immich, H. & Martini, H. (1969). Inzidenz seelischer Erkrankungen in Mannheim 1965. *Social Psychiatry*, **4**, 126–35.

Reimann H., Häfner, H. (1972). Psychische Erkrankungen alter Menschen in Mannheim. Eine Untersuchung der 'Konsultations-Inzidenz'. *Social Psychiatry*, **7**, 53–69.

Häfner, H. & Böker, W. (1973). Mentally disordered violent offenders. *Social Psychiatry*, **8**, 220–9.

Häfner, H. (1974). Der Einfluß von Umweltfaktoren auf die seelische Gesundheit. Ergebnisse, Möglichkeiten und Grenzen der Forschung. *Psychiatria Clinica*, **7**, 199–225.

Häfner, H., Moschel, G. & Ozek, M. (1977). Psychische Störungen bei türkischen Gastarbeitern. Eine prospektivepidemiologische Studie zur Untersuchung der Reaktion auf Einwanderung und partielle Anpassung. *Nervenarzt*, **48**, 268–75.

Häfner, H. (ed.) (1978). *Psychiatrische Epidemiologie*. Monographien aus dem Gesamtgebiete der Psychiatrie, Band 17. Berlin, Heidelberg & New York: Springer.

Häfner, H. (ed.) (1979). *Estimating Needs for Mental Health Care. A Contribution of Epidemiology*. Berlin, Heidelberg & New York: Springer.

Häfner, H. (1980). Psychiatrische Morbidität von Gastarbeitern in Mannheim. Epidemiologische Analyse einer Inanspruchnahmepopulation. *Nervenarzt*, **51**, 672–83.

Häfner, H. (1981). Der Krankheitsbegriff in der Psychiatrie. In *Standorte der Psychiatrie*, Band 2, *Zum umstrittenen psychiatrischen Krankheitsbegriff*, ed. R. Degwitz & H. Siedow, pp. 16–54. München, Wien & Baltimore: Urban & Schwarzenberg.

Häfner, H. & Klug, J. (1982). The impact of an expanding community mental health service on patterns of bed usage: evaluation of a four-year period of implementation. *Psychological Medicine*, **12**, 177–90.

Häfner, H. & Böker, W. (1982). Crimes of violence by mentally abnormal offenders. Cambridge: Cambridge University Press.

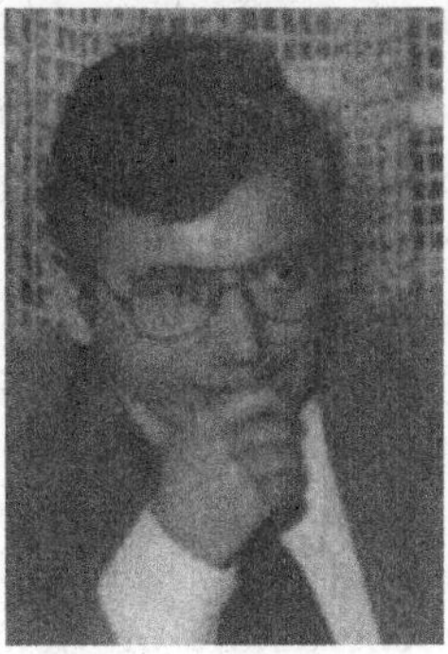

5 · ASSEN JABLENSKY

Personal background and professional experience

I was born in Sofia, Bulgaria, in 1940. After graduation from high school I studied medicine in Sofia between 1960 and 1966. My interest in psychiatry dates from the early years in medical school, where my teachers in the discipline were Academician G. Usunoff (1904–71), Professor N. Schipkowenski (1906–76) and Professor I. Temkov (present Director of the Department of Psychiatry). I acquired my postgraduate qualifications in psychiatry after a period of study in Bulgaria (1967–8) and in the United Kingdom (1968–9), where I worked as a registrar at the Maudsley Hospital in London with Professor M. Shepherd. After my return to Bulgaria, I was a research associate at the Institute of Sociology of the Bulgarian Academy of Sciences and a university lecturer in clinical psychiatry at the Medical Academy of Sofia. Since 1975 I have been a Senior Medical Officer with the Division of Mental Health, World Health Organisation, Geneva.

My interests and publications are in the fields of epidemiological psychiatry, cross-cultural psychiatry, research methodology, sociology of medicine and history of ideas. I have participated in a major survey of disability and levels of health in Bulgaria, in epidemiological studies of depressive illnesses and of general psychiatric morbidity in Bulgaria, in the WHO International Pilot Study of Schizophrenia, and in ongoing WHO-sponsored cross-cultural and epidemiological research in schizophrenia, depression and disability associated with mental disorder.

Assen Jablensky

Current status of psychiatry

An attempt to evaluate the current status of psychiatry is a formidable task which ought to be preceded by certain qualifications. The status of psychiatry as a practical activity (a 'helping profession') need not coincide with the status of psychiatry as a scientific field of inquiry. Furthermore, each of these two aspects of the discipline could be examined from different points of view: the present state may be compared to the past, the state of psychiatry may be compared to that of other medical disciplines, or the development of psychiatry may be compared in different cultures and societies. These different points of view are probably of equal relevance to the question 'Whither psychiatry?', but a comprehensive analysis encompassing them all would be an undertaking which surpasses both the scope of this essay and my capacity. I will therefore limit myself to a *selection of themes*, which in my view illustrate the current *problématique* of the discipline and are more or less peculiar to psychiatry. I will also attempt to enumerate significant current trends and developments, and venture a projection into the future.

In doing this, I deliberately narrow down my discussion on psychiatry as a professional discipline which is a sub-territory of the wider area of mental health. The latter is a loosely demarcated area of activities and concerns and a ground on which many disciplines and 'sectors' meet. The former, however, is a part of medicine which includes a body of theory, prescriptions about the rules for transmittal of established knowledge and for acquisition of new knowledge, and a set of rules about clinical practice, its organisation and regulation. The sequence of the discussion will, therefore, lead from the general paradigm within which psychiatry operates, through an attempted appraisal of the state of knowledge in the discipline, to issues of practical work. This convenient sequence does not, of course, imply the real existence of any kind of clear-cut hierarchy between these different levels.

Three characteristics of contemporary psychiatry strike me as prominent: (i) the insufficient attention paid by the discipline to its philosophical and value-oriented premises; (ii) the continuing ambiguities concerning the definition and boundaries of its subject-matter; and (iii) the gaps in knowledge and the relative immaturity of its theoretical apparatus.

Is a value-free psychiatry possible?

Psychiatry is a medical discipline. As such, it is embedded in the context of 'health care', a social sub-system which in turn belongs to the societal *superstructure*, in the Marxist sense of the term. The basic characteristics of the health care sub-system are determined by the nature of the socioeconomic base either directly – for example, through the general 'pull' effect of technological and scientific progress on the level which specific medical technologies occupy in the health system, or through class relations which determine the dominant mode of distribution of health care resources – or indirectly, through the mediation of other superstructure elements, such as ideology, law and the state. These relationships are complex and dynamic, and their analysis should avoid over-simplifications. Illich's *Medical Nemesis* (Illich, 1976) is an example of a skilful hypostasy of one particular aspect of the relationship of the socioeconomic base of the health care system, namely the technologisation of medicine, at the expense of the blurring of other, equally important phenomena and interactions.

The discipline of psychiatry is, of course, subject to the general influences of society which determine the structural attributes of health practice as a whole. These include resources, cost, methods of financing, investment policies (for example, investments in mental hospitals versus investments in community services), recruitment and social background of professionals, role and support of research and, perhaps most important, the mode of delivery, for example free-market medicine versus socialised health care. The position of psychiatry, however, exhibits certain specific features in addition which are less visible, though not altogether absent from other medical fields. The development of psychiatry, of course, depends on scientific advances in fields like neurochemistry, physiology, genetics, pharmacology, epidemiology and clinical science. Philosophical assumptions of a more general nature, however, play in psychiatry a greater and more immediate role than in other medical disciplines. Whatever psychiatrists profess, they deal with the human mind and behaviour and hence with those sensitive and value-laden domains of social reality where ideologically coloured images of 'human nature' influence the outlook of help-providers and help-seekers alike. Ideologically, man may be conceptualised as an instinctive, competitive and aggressive animal; as a mere envelope for genes, equipped with a cognitive computer which calculates the cost–benefit effect of 'altruistic' acts on the procreation of his DNA molecules; as a 'consumer' entitled to unrestricted 'pursuit of happiness'; or as a basically rational, affiliative being, capable of unlimited development in the process of social transformation of reality. Any of these diverse images of 'human nature' may find its reflection in different brands of psychiatric theory and practice.

The cultivation of a scotoma for the specific impact of ideological and philosophical assumptions on the historical development of the discipline of psychiatry would make it difficult to understand three important phenomena. First is the rise and fall of comprehensive theories which 'explain it all', for example psychoanalysis, learning theory, existential psychiatry and the recent excursions of sociobiology. Secondly, there is the oscillation and frequent polarisation of topic selection and orientation in psychiatric research, for example biological *or* social approaches, with little in the way of intermediate positions. And thirdly, there are the fluctuations in the self-definition and self-conceptualisation of the discipline, for example as a medical speciality dealing only with diseases and illnesses, or as a form of social engineering aimed at the improvement of the general level of 'mental health' of society.

The influence of philosophical assumptions and general societal values on psychiatry should be recognised as a fact, whether one regards it as a desirable or an undesirable fact. Even the particular variety of an empiricist and 'eclectic' orientation in psychiatry, which claims to be bound by nothing short of the pure Popperian criteria of science and fastidiously avoids philosophical speculation, is in real practice hardly untouched by ideology.

Turning now to the question of whether a value-free psychiatry is possible, it may be of interest to examine whether it carries different implications from those of analogous questions, like whether a value-free surgery is possible. Few would search for deep-seated principles underlying routine surgery, yet it is known that appendectomies, for instance, are performed twice as frequently per 1,000 population in the USA compared to Britain and that this difference cannot be explained by the relative incidence of perforated appendix in the two countries. The reasons for the different behaviour of appendices and surgeons have probably something to do with societal values, for example with prevalent ideas about 'health conditions' requiring intervention, with the expectations of the clientele, and possibly with surgeons' views about remuneration. Over-demand and over-supply, or under-demand and under-supply, the type and the quality of medical care all reflect societal values and the hidden forces which shape them. In this sense neither psychiatry, nor surgery, nor any other medical discipline can be value-free.

Psychiatry, however, is value-bound in yet another sense, because it cannot afford to be 'soulless'. Psychiatry can hardly survive as a discipline if, in the encounters with the patient, it treats him as a mere assembly of enzymes, neuronal circuits, stimulus–response sequences or symptoms assessed in a standardised manner to provide input to a computerised diagnostic programme. The essence of the practice of psychiatry lies in skills which aim to relate all these different aspects of the human being to the totality of experience, to the here and now of the patient's life and to his personality as a 'set of social relationships' (Marx, 1844). This, of course, should be the ethos of good medical practice in any discipline, but it is *technically* pivotal to psychiatry. The historical evolution of psychiatry as a discipline can be judged on the merits of *whether*, *how* and *for whom* such skills are applied (or not applied) and this is a question which can be answered only with reference to value-oriented criteria. Such criteria cannot be generated within the discipline only. The recognition of this fact may eventually contribute to the development of a social epistemology and a deontology of psychiatry, leading to a systematic examination of its premises, its links with philosophical and humanistic concerns, empirical science and societal praxis.

Viability of definitions of mental illness and mental health

The need for a systematic exploration of the epistemological and axiological premises of contemporary psychiatry is further emphasised by the fact that psychiatry has been the target of militant critique and loud propaganda with potentially damaging implications for the treatment of many people who might seek and benefit from good psychiatric care. This situation can be seen as a modern exacerbation and acting out of ambiguities which have been fellow-travellers of the discipline of psychiatry since its emergence as a form of professional activity and scientific inquiry. The ambiguities concern the definition of the concepts of 'mental illness' and 'mental health', and the question of the legitimacy of the medical handling of problems which – in the view of those who challenge the *raison d'être* of psychiatry – properly belong either to somatic medicine or to the domains of morality, theology or social relations. None of the varied view-points in the anti-psychiatry debate of the last decade is entirely new; one is reminded, for example, of Kant's contention that judgements on matters of sanity should be the prerogative of the 'philosophical faculty' (Kant, 1872). None of the issues involved in the debate need to be limited to psychiatry: the epistemological and deontological problems involved in the definition of health and disease in general are no less formidable than those related to the subject-matter of psychiatry. Even so, the anti-psychiatric critique capitalises on psychiatry's reluctance to examine its own premises and to put its own theoretical house in order. The issues are being further confused by the currently fashionable theorising about a 'medical model of disease' as contrasted to a 'sociological model of deviance'. This is a pseudo-dilemma, because a search for evidence of the existence of an entity, such as a single and monolithic 'medical model', would be in vain, not least of all in psychiatry, where the parallel recognition of sociogenic causation and organic determinism has been part and parcel of the dialectics of its development since the early nineteenth century. This pseudo-dilemma, however, is often presented as a forced choice and as a watershed dividing the 'bad' and 'good' camps within the discipline.

The truly scientific concept of disease has always incorporated an implicit or explicit social dimension. In general medicine the early work of Virchow – who, ironically, became later associated with cellular pathology only – or in psychiatry of Korsakoff – who coined the term 'social psychiatry' (Melekhov, 1975) – are among the many examples. Whatever the heuristic value of recent concepts like deviance, labelling and attribution, they are unlikely to provide either a basis or a rationale for a re-definition of the concept of mental illness, though they are of definite help in the conceptualisation of various forms of behaviour related to the phenomena of mental disorders. This does not mean that the current psychiatric concept of mental illness, formulated in the course of the nineteenth century, is immutable. There is no doubt that it has already undergone considerable evolution and refinement. By and large, however, it has remained within the confines of the same basic paradigm which had found an expression in Jaspers' (1963) tripartite synthetic definition dividing the abnormal mental phenomena into accompaniments of somatic morbid *processes*, abnormal *reactions* and 'unwanted variations' of *development*. No evidence has come forth to challenge seriously the validity of this concept; on the contrary, a body of supportive data has been accumulated in its favour, including, in particular, the weighty testimony of cross-cultural observations. The present paradigm of mental illness may become obsolete some day, but until the arrival of a better replacement, it seems to function reasonably well. To sum up, I believe that the medical definition of mental illness (incorporating also a behavioural and social dimension) is viable and universally applicable.

Not so with mental health. The concepts of mental illness and mental health are of a different nature and the one is not the reciprocal value of the other. Leaving aside instances when the term 'mental health' is used as a collective noun for various disciplines and practical activities, the concept of mental health as an attribute of man is as ambiguous as the generic concept of health. Attempts to operationalise and measure positive mental health as different from the mere absence of illness have produced either trivial results or lists of desirable traits and behaviours reflecting the characteristics of particular social groups or cultures (a critical review of the problem has been provided by Herzlich, 1973). In my view, the concept of mental health has an entirely different status from the concept of mental illness. Mental health is a value-concept, while mental illness is not. Normative elements predominate in the former, descriptive in the latter. A corollary of this would be the inherent historic and cultural relativity, within certain limits, of the mental health ideal. Unfortunately, the fact that mental health and mental illness belong to two different classes of concept is frequently overlooked, with the result either that the notion of mental health is discussed as 'unscientific' or that vague references to some elusive entity which defies a closer definition tend to proliferate. A more fruitful approach might be one based on medical anthropology, which could systematically explore and bring into focus the elements of the mental health ideal implicit in different cultures and societies.

The status of knowledge and the theoretical apparatus of psychiatry

Psychiatric research in the last decade or so has been characterised by cumulative increases in knowledge and not by the emergence of any radically new ideas or of a major discovery which could revolutionise the field. The increment of knowledge has been achieved mainly through refinements of techniques, confirmation or rejection of earlier ideas and, more generally, by building upon foundations laid earlier. My list of more significant achievements would include, for instance, the wide recognition of the need to standardise and operationalise assessment methods and diagnostic criteria, the increased knowledge about side-effects of psychotropic drugs, the accumulation of evidence that basic forms of the major psychoses can be reliably recognised in different cultures, the application of epidemiological approaches to the study of mental disorder in children and the swing of the pendulum towards high-quality research in biological psychiatry whose outcome is yet to be seen. To this, I would add the generally improved methodological standards of published studies and the emergence of original psychiatric research in many developing countries.

Yet the absence of major milestones is conspicuous. Psychiatric research has not been able to emulate achievements of the order of Goldberger's studies on pellagra (Goldberger, 1914) or the more recent work on Kuru

(Gajdusek & Zigas, 1957). The net progress in our understanding of such major problems as the aetiology and pathogenesis of the major psychoses, of the interrelations between genetic and environmental factors in human behaviour, and of the mechanisms underlying the dementing illnesses of middle and old age has been extremely modest. A recent review of the 'successes of prevention' (Fielding, 1978) quotes some impressive advances in several fields of medicine, but none in psychiatry (except for a brief mention of secondary prevention in phenylketonuria under the rubric 'congenital metabolic diseases').

Progress in psychiatric knowledge meets obstacles at different levels. First there is an epistemological 'sound barrier' to be overcome. The complexity of the phenomena of mental life and their multiple determination present an inherent difficulty which not infrequently leads into the trap of reductionism, be it in the form of a search for a 'mad molecule' (to use J. P. Donleavy's phrase) or in the form of a sociological 'labelling' theory. I was impressed, for example, by the way a scientist, distinguished for his pioneering work on brain opioid peptides, recently described in a discussion the logic behind modern biological research: 'Now that we have a fundamental mechanism consisting of a specific receptor site and an endorphin, we must start 'building' hypothetical diseases around it' (E. J. Simon, personal communication). The intellectual attractiveness of this model of research which predicts attributes of disease from established characteristics of a basic biological mechanism is powerful, but its application in psychiatry is not yet within reach nor is its applicability in principle unequivocally clear. There is a profound lack of basic knowledge about the mechanisms of the mind, in spite of the steady progress of the neurosciences. The phenomena which interest the psychiatrist can be stratified on three levels of organisation: biological–organic, psychological–experiential and social–behavioural. A theory which aims to account for complex disturbances like schizophrenia must make certain assumptions about the nature of interrelations between different levels of organisation. Such assumptions are at present of a very general nature and they are too weak to generate significant hypotheses for empirical research. It is perhaps too early to expect a dialectical 'leap' to a new synthesis of previously unrelated and often conflicting facts.

The second kind of obstacle is of a more mundane kind and involves social and economic factors. Generally, psychiatric research is an astonishingly low priority on the books of funding agencies, and the volume of adequately supported, technically sound mental health research in the world is very small in proportion to the size, severity and intractability of the problems it is supposed to tackle. If research is the 'lifeline of medicine' (Kornberg, 1976), then the survival of psychiatry depends on a very thin thread. This situation has a direct bearing on the selection and self-selection of research workers ready to commit themselves to psychiatry. For many of them, the choice may have to be made at the expense of a clinical career and the main factor in the decision may be the intellectual appeal and social prestige of the work rather than the income derived from it. Although the number of intelligent young people taking up a research career in psychiatry seems to be increasing, it remains small in comparison with other areas of biomedical research. Limited funds, the small number of talented people determined enough to choose psychiatric research as a vocation and the modest yield of such research failing to capture the imagination of administrators form a vicious circle which retards the growth of knowledge.

A third problem affecting progress in research is the lack of effective communication. This is illustrated, for example, by the striking 'ethnocentricity' of the references usually quoted in publications (this phenomenon seems to be particularly marked in British and American psychiatric research). Another example is the almost total ignorance in the West about developments in psychiatric research in Eastern Europe* and, to a lesser extent, in the developing countries. Scientific exchanges have, indeed, increased rapidly in the last few years, but they cannot replace the role of a widely read and prestigious psychiatric journal. Nevertheless, it is precisely the most widely read journals which are curiously ineffective in ensuring wide international participation and, intentionally or not, perpetuate a linguistic bias which usually coincides to some extent with a geopolitical area. In view of this trend, I believe that a wise, balanced and forward-looking editorial policy of the leading psychiatric journals could be an invaluable, internationally important stimulus for research, if pursued with vigour and persistence.

Significant trends in psychiatric practice

In the last decade, psychiatry has shown a definite trend towards a closer co-operation with a number of other medical fields. This, in my opinion,

* The impression of the author is that, on the average, Eastern European psychiatrists are better informed about research in the West than their Western counterparts about research in Eastern Europe. The asymmetry can hardly be explained by a language barrier, since practically all psychiatric journals published in Eastern Europe include English, and sometimes French, language summaries.

is perhaps the most important development, and evidence of such convergence can be found in many countries. General practitioners (or doctors in equivalent positions) are increasingly interested in the psychological aspects of morbidity in the community, and many of them are now engaged in the treatment of large numbers of people presenting with psychiatric problems. The fact that the major share of non-psychotic mental morbidity is found within general practice populations (who also appear to be the larger group of consumers of the psychotropic products of the pharmaceutical industry) is by now well documented in several parts of the world, and if any revision is to be made of the prevalence figures obtained more than a decade ago by Shepherd, Cooper, Brown & Kalton (1966), it is likely to be a revision upwards. It has become clear that the problems of these patients fit poorly the conventional psychiatric nosology, that lucid guidelines for the rational treatment and management of such cases are lacking and that neither general practitioners nor psychiatrists are adequately prepared to manage them. This realisation has obvious implications for research, for medical and psychiatric training and for the organisation of services. An example of organisational change is the trend in several Eastern European countries and in the USSR to allocate psychiatrists to primary health care teams, for instance in general polyclinics serving defined catchment areas (although such areas would also have a psychiatric outpatient centre). In other health care systems, a response to the problem has been the provision of 'refresher' training in psychiatry for general practitioners.

Another important fact is the discovery (supported by epidemiological data) that the burden of psychiatric illness on the general health services is as large, or even larger, in the developing countries. On a global scale, this is perhaps the most serious practical problem facing psychiatry today. The widening gap between the rapidly increasing populations at risk for mental disorders and the slow increase (or possibly decrease) in the number of skilled mental health workers is of a magnitude precluding obvious solutions. The search for new approaches and solutions constitutes an area which offers practically limitless opportunities for innovation, as it is now clear that the conventional models of mental health care are not practicable.

In more narrowly defined fields, the growing interaction between psychiatry and other medical disciplines is another current trend of potential significance. Fields like endocrinology, cardiology, orthopaedics, occupational medicine and prevention of tropical diseases offer unexpected prospects for the application of psychiatric skills and research techniques. If this trend finds further support, the old maxim that major advances in knowledge are often made at the borderline between disciplines may receive refreshing confirmation.

The positive trend of a diffusion of psychiatric skills toward other domains of medicine and health care contrasts with the state of stagnation in the realm of institutional psychiatry. It is true that a number of mental hospitals in different parts of the world have been transformed from asylums into 'therapeutic communities', or at least into decent institutions where treatment is given. However, in spite of the hopes raised almost two decades ago by the 'psycho-pharmacological revolution', the majority of mental hospitals have remained more or less untouched by innovation; they remain understaffed and overcrowded, operating at standards of care which in most countries would be totally unacceptable in somatic medicine. The mental hospital is no longer the pivot of psychiatry, but in the eyes of the public it is still a trademark of the discipline. The neglected hospital, forgotten in the backwater of the discipline, hardly improves public attitude toward psychiatry.

One of the dramatic events in the last decade has been the relatively sudden and rapid discharge of large numbers of so-called 'chronic' patients into unprepared and frequently inhospitable communities. Such steps were hailed as unqualified progress until the moment of realisation that the burden of chronic disability associated with mental disorder did not decrease but only shifted its locus. There is perhaps better knowledge now about the types of environment in which mentally disabled people can function reasonably well, but the current provision of community facilities designed on such principles is far from adequate. Disability prevention and rehabilitation, in my view, make up an area where policies adopted and enforced at the social system level may exercise a considerable impact. My own impressions are that in the area of community-based rehabilitation facilities the socialist countries are moving faster than the West and have adopted more comprehensive policies.

A comment should perhaps be devoted to the unfulfilled promises of psychiatry. The missionary zeal with which claims were made in the past about psychiatry's calling to solve social problems, ranging from control of violence to prevention of armed conflicts among nations through psychiatric counselling of political leaders, has almost vanished. More realistic applications of psychiatric knowledge to the social field, like the prevention of traffic accidents or advice to urban planners and industrial managers, have rarely produced more than trivial recommendations. Short of extravagant claims, there is nothing intrinsically wrong in the search for new and useful social roles for psychiatry. The state of knowledge, however, and the pitifully small intellectual and material resources devoted to serious research in such 'applied' fields limit at present its role as a medical discipline contributing to social development.

To conclude my remarks on the present state of psychiatry, I should like to mention some concerns regarding the teaching of psychiatry and behavioural sciences in medical schools. The inadequate number of hours devoted to psychiatry and behavioural disciplines has often been deplored in many countries. However, a simple increase in the number of hours for psychiatry and related sciences is unlikely to remove what Kabanov & Tzaregorodtzev (1979) have called 'the danger of biological reductionism in the training and work of the physician'. One approach that could prove effective to counteract this danger is the systematic integration of elements of psychological medicine into the teaching programmes of other medical disciplines, but one wonders how many medical schools might be prepared to take such a minor step which would indicate a major change of attitude.

The postgraduate training of psychiatrists generally suffers, in my view, from two deficiencies. One is the relative neglect, especially in recent years, of the teaching of general psychopathology. Whatever the expansion of curricula to cover new subjects like ethology or human communication, psychopathology remains the basic clinical tool to be mastered by the psychiatrist. The second deficiency is the inadequate teaching of epidemiology and social medicine, a deficiency which is perhaps implicated in the resistance of psychiatrists to learning from general public health experience. Although the psychiatric profession in most parts of the world includes a minority of exceptionally well trained and able people, the average psychiatrist is, on the whole, perhaps less competent in his discipline than other medical specialists in theirs, the distance between good average and barely tolerable skills in clinical psychiatry being smaller than in other fields.

Future prospects of psychiatry

My main feeling about the present state of psychiatry is perhaps one of discontent and impatience with its progress. I see no reason for complacency about the current state of affairs in the face of widespread and severe problems for which we have no solution. The growing iceberg of chronic disability, the psychological illness or distress associated with an increasing range of occupational and daily living situations, the spectre of dementia affecting a rising proportion of mankind as populations grow older, are all real challenges for society as a whole and for the mental health disciplines in particular. These are clear priorities for research and for eventual preventive programmes, in both East and West (for example, Schmidt & Snezhnevskij, 1978; Eisenberg, 1977). In the Third World the overwhelming needs at present are in the area of services and training of personnel (WHO, 1975), but progress in these areas will require the steady support of epidemiology, clinical psychopharmacology and evaluation methodology. There is evidently a full programme for psychiatry, and it is difficult to find realistic grounds either for predictions of a gradual dissolution of psychiatry into neurology and social counselling (Fuller Torrey, 1974), or for negative Utopias of the 'brave new world' type.

I believe that psychiatry is slowly growing into maturity. While the basic structure of the discipline is unlikely to change much in the coming decades, two possibilities, one of a 'developmental spurt' and one of an indefinitely retarded growth, seem to be equally open. Which of the two possibilities will become a reality depends on a multitude of factors, of which only a few are under the control of the psychiatric profession. The volume of material and societal support which psychiatry needs for a take-off, away from its present state of poverty and low productivity, will depend on the realisation, or lack of realisation, by decision-makers and public opinion of the socially useful role that the discipline has to play in meeting the demands posed by a rapidly changing environment and lifestyle. Scientific progress within psychiatry will probably depend to a great extent on the 'carry-over' and stimulation effects of discoveries made in basic research and in 'borderline' zones between disciplines. The practical application of any advances in psychiatric knowledge, however, will ultimately depend on the ability of psychiatry to permeate general health care, and establish for itself both scientific respectability and acceptance as a humanising presence and influence.

Questions and answers

1. In view of your personal experience and your views on the importance of sociocultural factors in determining the theory and practice of psychiatry, could you comment on the similarities and differences characterising the subject in Eastern and Western Europe?

Undoubtedly, there are both similarities and differences caused by a variety of factors related to historical development and tradition, socio-economic patterns and the general characteristics of the discipline.

Perhaps the level at which moost similarities can be found is that of the *operational tools* of the psychiatrist: diagnostic and therapeutic techniques, research methods and clinical concepts. Variation at this level seems to originate mainly in the existence of different schools giving more emphasis to one or another class of techniques or research methods, rather than in the more global differences between countries or groups of countries. At the level of *theory*, the situation is more complex. Cross-fertilisation does occur, and one could quote as examples the influence of Pavlovian concepts on the development of behaviour therapy or of Luria's ideas on the approach to understanding the psychological sequelae of brain damage in the West, and of Selye's stress theory on clinical thinking and research in East European countries. However, the diffusion of theories with philosophical and ideological implications, like psychoanalysis, is a different matter. While a number of problems raised by psychoanalytical thinking, like the role of unconscious mental mechanisms, have been recognised as important areas for scientific inquiry by psychiatrists in Eastern Europe (Bassine, Rojnov & Rojnova, 1973), the philosophical generalisations of psychoanalysis, implying a particular *Weltanschauunng*, a historically dated view on the nature of man and society, have found no following there because they do not correspond to the *praxis* and values of society as a whole.

There are quite important differences between psychiatry in Eastern and Western Europe at the level of organisation of services and delivery of care. Psychiatry in the East European countries is embedded within a system of socialised medicine and health care, and private practice is either non-existent, or has a very limited place. In the framework of the present system of psychiatric care delivery in most East European countries, the mental hospital has a less central role to play than in many West European countries and for many years the emphasis has been placed on outpatient and community care. The principles of social and community psychiatry as an alternative to institutional psychiatry have been extensively developed as an 'integration of the social and individual clinical points of view' (Gannushkin, 1924) in the Soviet Union after the October Revolution, and influenced the reform and development of mental health services in Eastern Europe in the post-war period, well before the term 'social psychiatry' became current in the West. One of the results of this pattern of service development is the considerably smaller size of the 'long-stay' population in psychiatric institutions in East European countries by comparison with several West European countries, even allowing for the recent significant rise of discharges. In an epidemiological study in an urban catchment area in Bulgaria, in which my colleagues and I were involved (Temkov, Jablensky & Boyadjieva, 1975), methods of case-finding and rate computation were similar to those employed in a British–US study. While the overall prevalence rates were found to be of a comparable magnitude, the number of long-stay patients per 1,000 in the Bulgarian catcchment area was 5.6 times lower than in the British, and 9.5 times lower than in the US area.

The emphasis on outpatient care is accompanied by a parallel emphasis on industrial rehabilitation, as already mentioned. These are, in my view, important assets of East European psychiatry which are likely to determine its future development.

The psychiatric scene in Western Europe is more difficult to describe in terms of general pattern and trends because of marked differences in the 'style' of psychiatry and in systems of care between, for example, countries like the United Kingdom and Italy, or the Scandinavian countries and Spain or Portugal. I think that the movement toward community care is a trend which can be found almost everywhere but the problems it encounters at the level of implementation, for example difficulties in financing and the strong incentives for psychiatrists to devote themselves to individual therapy, normally on a private basis, illustrate the point about the socioeconomic base which I made above.

2. Could you elaborate on your expressed opinion about the potential value of medical anthropology for mental health?

I believe that anthropology can provide a complementary frame of reference to medical thinking which would increase our understanding of the cultural context of health and disease, and forge links (very few exist so far) with epidemiological research, as has been the case with investigations on neurological and dementing illnesses in West New Guinea (Gajdusek, 1977). In my view, this is a methodologically fascinating approach. This approach has not been sufficiently extended to the study of mental disorders in different societies, although isolated examples can be found in the literature on transcultural psychiatry (for example, Burton-Bradley, 1975). So far medical anthropology has concentrated predominantly on disease and on so-called primitive human communities. The implicit or explicit concepts of mental health as a desirable psychological state or way of relating to the world in different cultures have been little explored, especially in industrialised societies and in societies in transition. Psychiatric epidemiologists developing methods for cross-cultural application have not yet found much help from their anthropological colleagues.

As a primarily 'understanding', rather than a 'counting', discipline, anthropology and related social sciences could provide hypotheses which psychiatry cannot generate alone. It would be of interest, for example, to study the formation of the self-image in different cultures; the 'modal' personality in different societies or the threshold of resistance to stressful events in relation to cultural values. I think that Bateson's 'double-bind' hypothesis (Bateson, Jackson, Haley & Weakland, 1956) is likely to be refuted, but it is nevertheless an example of the stimulating effect that anthropological thinking can have on psychiatric research. Generally, the dialogue between the two disciplines should be more intensive than it has been up to the present.

3. What practical steps could be taken to implement the 'wise, balanced and forward-looking editorial policy of leading psychiatric journals' to which you refer?

Examples of *possible* steps could be: (i) the adoption of an explicit policy of stimulating contributions from outside one's own cultural area; (ii) the recruitment of reviewers with wide cultural experience and knowledge of languages; (iii) the commissioning of review articles which cover significant research published in less accessible languages; (iv) a willingness to invest in translation, thereby encouraging potential authors who find it difficult to write in the language of the journal; and (v) the establishing of co-operation with psychiatric journals in different parts of the world and the publication of joint issues.

References

Bassine, P., Rojnov, V. & Rojnova, M. (1973). Ce que nous pensons de la psychoanalyse. *L'Évolution Psychiatrique*, 3, 387–404.

Bateson, G., Jackson, D. D., Haley, J. & Weakland, J. H. (1956). Towards a theory of schizophrenia. *Behavioural Science*, 1, 4. (Reprinted in Bateson, G., (1973). *Steps to an Ecology of Mind*. London: Paladin.)

Burton-Bradley, B. G. (1975). *Stone Age Crisis. A Psychiatric Appraisal*. Nashville: Vanderbilt University Press.

Eisenberg, L. (1977). The social imperatives of medical research. *Science*, 198, 1105–10.

Fielding, J. E. (1978). Successes of prevention. *Milbank Memorial Fund Quarterly/Health and Society*, 56, 3, 274–302.

Fuller Torrey, E. (1974). *The Death of Psychiatry*. New York & Baltimore: Penguin Books Inc.

Gajdusek, D. C. (1977). Urgent opportunistic observations: the study of changing, transient and disappearing phenomena of medical interest in disrupted primitive human communities. In *Health and Disease in Tribal Societies*, Ciba Foundation Symposium 49. Amsterdam, Oxford & New York: Elsevier, Excerpta Medica, North-Holland.

Gajdusek, D. C. & Zigas, V. (1957). Degenerative disease of the central nervous system in New Guinea: the endemic appearance of Kuru in the native population. *New England Journal of Medicine*, 257, 974–8.

Gannushkin, P. B. (1924). *Psychiatry: its Objectives, Scope and Teaching* (Russian) Moscow. (Quoted after Melekhov, D. E. (1975).

Goldberger, J. (1914). The etiology of pellagra. *Public Health Reports* **29** (26), 1683.

Herzlich, C. (1973). *Health and Illness. A Social Psychological Analysis*. London & New York: Academic Press.

Illich, I. (1976). *Limits to Medicine. Medical Nemesis: The Expropriation of Health*. New York & Baltimore: Penguin Books Inc.

Jaspers, K. (1963). *General Psychopathology*. Translated by J. Hoenig & M. W. Hamilton. Manchester University Press.

Kabanov, M. M. & Tzaregorodtzev, G. I. (1979). Medicine and psychology. *Vestnik Akademii Medizinskih Nunk SSSR (Journal of the Academy of Medical Sciences of USSR*), 5, 45–51.

Kant, I. (1872) *Anthropologie in pragmatischer Hinsicht* (2. Auflage). Berlin: Kirchmann.

Kornberg, A. (1976). Research, the lifeline of medicine. *New England Journal of Medicine*, **294**, 22, 1212–16.

Marx, K. (1844). Ökonomisch-philosophische Manuskripte, in Marx-Engels Studienansgabe, Band II. Frankfurt am Main, Fischer Verlag, 1966.

Melekhov, D. E. (1975). P. B. Gannushkin and the development of social psychiatry in USSR. *Zhurnal nevropatologii i psihiatrii im S. S. Korsakova*, 75, 4, 583–6.

Schmidt, E. V. & Snezhnevskij, A. V. (1976). Research in neuropathology and psychiatry. *Vestnik Akademii Medizinskih Nunk SSSR (Journal of the Academy of Medical Sciences of USSR*), 12, 57–60.

Shepherd, M., Cooper, B., Brown, A. C. & Kalton G. W. (1966) *Psychiatric Illness in General Practice*. London: Oxford University Press.

Temkov, I., Jablensky, A. & Boyadjieva, M. (1975). Use of reported prevalence data in cross-national comparisons of psychiatric morbidity. *Socijalna Psihijatrija*, 3, 111–17.

World Health Organisation (1975). *Organisation of Mental Health Services in Developing Countries*. Sixteenth Report of the WHO Expert Committee on Mental Health, Technical Report Series no. 564. Geneva: World Health Organisation.

Select bibliography

Dimitrov, Ch., & Jablensky, A. (1967). Nietzsche und Freud. *Zsch. Psychosomat. Med. u. Psychoanalyse*, 13, 282–98.

Jablensky, A. & Oschavkov, J. (1975). Health and disability in a total population. In *Health, Medicine, Society*, ed. M. Sokolowska, J. Holowka & A. Ostrowska, pp.51–8. Reidel Publ. Comp.

Jablensky, A. & Sartorius, N. (1975). Culture and schizophrenia. In *On the Origin of the Schizophrenic Psychoses*, ed. H. M. Van Praag, pp.99–124. Amsterdam: De Erven Bohn BV.

Jablensky, A. & Sartorius, N. (1975). Culture and schizophrenia (editorial). *Psychological Medicine*, 5, 113–24.

Jablensky, A. (1976). Personality disorders and their relationship to illness and social deviance. *Psychiatric Annals*, 6, 8.

Jablensky, A. (1977). Racism, apartheid and mental health. *World Health* (December), pp.16–21.

Jablensky, A. (1978). The need for standardisation of psychiatric assessment. The epidemiological point of view. *Acta psychiat. belg.* 78, 549–58.

Sartorius, N., Jablensky, A. & Shapiro, R. (1977). Two-year follow-up of the patients included in the WHO International Pilot Study of Schizophrenia, *Psychological Medicine*, 7, 529–41.

Sartorius, N., Jablensky, A. & Shapiro, R. (1978). Cross-cultural differences in the short-term prognosis of schizophrenic psychoses. *Schizophrenia Bulletin*, 4, 102–13.

Sheldrick, C., Jablensky, A., Sartorius, N. & Shepherd, M. (1977). Schizophrenia succeeded by affective illness: catamnestic study and statistical enquiry. *Psychological Medicine*, 7, 619–24.

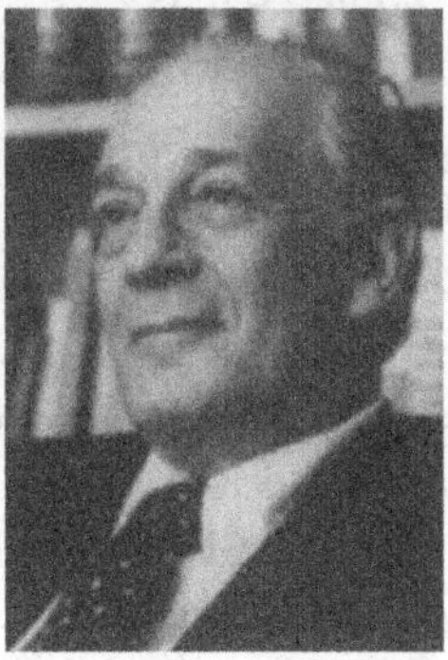

6 · SEYMOUR KETY

Personal background and professional experience

I was born, reared and educated in Philadelphia and by the time I reached adolescence had experienced a number of environmental influences which Anne Roe found with unusual frequency in her classical studies of the lives of biological and natural scientists. I was the first born and, for my first ten years, the only child. My father died when I was twelve and my mother's four sisters and brother shared their home with us. Although financial problems were present, so were books, great music and lively discussion. When I was seven, I was struck by a car and spent nearly a year in hospital and at home recovering from the injuries. During that time I read voraciously, particularly about science, and afterward compensated for my handicap in sports with a consuming interest in chemistry, satisfied by many hours spent after school in a constantly expanding basement laboratory. What might have become a one-sided education was rounded out with Latin, Greek and philosophy in an unusual high school.

My medical training was not to prepare me for practice but for biomedical research, which presented many interfaces of chemistry with biology and medicine. Indeed, my first research, begun as a medical student, was on the role of the citrate ion in the disposition of lead and its application to the treatment of lead poisoning. When I completed medical school I married Josephine Gross, who in the 40 years of our marriage has shared my work and decisions, gracefully adapting her career as a paediatrician to mine in the moves we decided to make.

This essay should properly be entitled 'A non-psychiatrist on psychiatry', since I am not a psychiatrist. For the past 30 years, however, I have devoted myself to psychiatric research, and two academic institutions have appointed me Professor of Psychiatry, identifying me in a generous synecdoche with the field as a whole.

My postdoctoral training was in circulatory and respiratory physiology with Joseph Aub, Carl Schmidt and Julius Comroe, and my involvement with psychiatry began with the cerebral circulation and the attached brain. Just as the brain is nourished and sustained by its circulation, so, in turn, is the discipline of psychiatry dependent on the sciences of the brain for its sustenance. That self-evident observation is not in contradiction with another equally valid one, that there is much more to the brain than the cerebral circulation and much more to psychiatry than the brain.

I joined Carl Schmidt's laboratory in 1942, attracted by his studies of the blood flow through the brain of the monkey, and was fortunate enough to participate in the measurements he was making of cerebral oxygen and glucose utilisation in these animals under deep and light anesthesia and during convulsions. Important as those studies were, however, I became engrossed in the possibility of deriving such knowledge about the human brain.

Just as the brain is unique among organs for its complexity, so the human brain is unique in its versatility and capacity, its ability to think and imagine, to experience profound emotions and to describe to the observer the results of its inner processes. It is the human brain also that falls prey to serious disorders of these functions and for which no comparable animal models exist. To study the metabolism of the human brain while engaged in those functions and experiences might teach us something about the underlying processes, and its study in disease might be of benefit to those suffering from neurological or mental disorders. The surgical procedures we were employing for the direct measurements in the monkey were out of the question in man and I set about to devise an indirect approach that could comfortably be applied to man under physiological conditions. Fick, Krogh and Bohr had developed expressions to describe the exchange of oxygen between the circulating blood and body tissues, but to measure metabolism it would be necessary to invoke processes that were independent of oxygen consumption. Such processes would be those involved in the exchange and uptake of diffusible but non-metabolised substances. I derived equations to describe the changing distribution of an inert gas between blood and cerebral tissues as they approached equilibrium and, utilising these, it was eventually possible to quantify the overall circulation and metabolism of the human brain.

Among the first disorders to be studied with the newly developed technique was schizophrenia, but in that condition no difference from normal was found for the circulation or oxygen utilisation of the brain as a whole. It was suggested that more subtle biochemical processes than energy metabolism were involved in schizophrenia and that, if changes in energy metabolism did indeed occur, they were restricted to certain regions and did not become apparent in the organ as a whole. Ten years elapsed before we were able to measure circulation in the small regions throughout the brain.

It was in the studies on schizophrenia that I first saw the temporary but remarkable restoration in the thinking and affect of some schizophrenics under the influence of sodium amytal narcosis. I was impressed that a drug could produce such dramatic effects, which suggested that biochemical processes on which a drug could act were responsible for the psychotic symptoms.

These studies had come to the attention of Robert Felix, Director of the newly founded National Institute of Mental Health in Bethesda, and in 1951 he invited me to join that Institute as its first Scientific Director. It was then that my commitment to psychiatric research began. For one who was challenged by the problem of mental illness, yet recognised that the magnitude of the problem was matched by our ignorance about it, what better opportunity existed than to plan and develop a research programme broad enough to examine the problem of mental illness in all of its complexities? We would need research at the clinical level, of course, but for that to be meaningful there was the greater need for considerably more fundamental knowledge in the sciences of brain and behaviour to provide the foundations of rational and plausible clinical research. I could think of no better investment of the new and unprecedented resources placed at my disposal than using them to establish a broad programme of fundamental research representing all of the disciplines on which psychiatry depends. Over the next few years laboratories were established in socio-environmental studies, neurophysiology, neurochemistry and chemical pharmacology. Under the aegis of the Neurological Institute, whose research programme I was also charged with organising, laboratories of neuroanatomy and biophysics were added. In concert with Robert Cohen, who had been appointed Director of Clinical Investigations in the Mental Health Institute, a large laboratory of psychology was organised representing a wide spectrum of experimental, developmental and clinical aspects of the field.

The resources made available at that time of great public appreciation and support of research, and the commitment not to make conspicuous relevance a desideratum, rendered it possible to recruit a number of established scientists of distinction and an even larger cohort of young investigators of great promise. In the 30 years that have elapsed, that promise has been amply fulfilled.

The responsibilities of Scientific Director did not consume all of my energies and it was possible to establish a small laboratory in which I could continue some research on cerebral circulation and metabolism. To that laboratory came Louis Sokoloff, who had worked with me at the University of Pennsylvania, and, for varying periods of time, William Landau, Lewis Rowland, Niels Lassen, Cesare Fieschi and Martin Reivich. It was found that although the nitrous oxide technique had been of value in the study of states in which a generalised change in blood flow or metabolism in the brain was involved, the complexity of the brain and the localisation of function within it demanded techniques capable of examining its circulation and metabolism in more minute detail. After some unsuccessful attempts to study the clearance of radioactive inert gas injected into the parenchyma of the brain, I remembered an equation I had developed just before coming to Bethesda which described the accumulation of an inert, diffusible substance locally, in terms of the perfusion prevailing at that site. We used a radioactive inert gas and made our first autoradiograms from frozen sections cut with a bandsaw. Later, the use of a non-gaseous tracer and sectioning with a microtome simplified the autoradiography. These techniques gave satisfactory visualisations of blood flow, which was usually well correlated with neuronal activity, but it was not until Sokoloff worked out the dynamics of deoxyglucose accumulation and demonstrated its close coupling with glucose metabolism and neuronal activity that the means of mapping glucose metabolism and the closely correlated levels of functional activity throughout the brain became available. This technique has been of inestimable value to the fundamental neurosciences. Positron-emission tomography makes it applicable to clinical problems where it will undoubtedly become a major contribution to diagnosis and research.

The basic and clinical programmes for intramural research at the National Institute of Mental Health had been organised independently and were pursuing their separate and, for the most part, divergent paths. By 1956 a number of investigators, whose interests lay in the interface between the basic neurobiological sciences and clinical psychiatric problems, particularly the major psychoses, had joined the Intramural Program. They established a new collaborative group designated the Laboratory of Clinical Science. By that time also the basic research programme was fully staffed, I was eager to involve myself more in research and less in administration, and the psychiatric implications of the new knowledge in the neurosciences attracted me. I was allowed to move from the position of Scientific Director to that of Chief of the Laboratory of Clinical Science.

What were these new and promising implications that attracted many of us? It was not the numerous enthusiastic claims that were being made regarding abnormal proteins, metabolites or toxic factors in the blood or urine of schizophrenic patients, which lacked plausibility and did not survive replication. Rather, it was a number of less spectacular but more credible observations with more remote relevance, observations that suggested that the synapses of the brain, like those in the periphery, were chemically mediated switches rather than electrical junctions. Acetylcholine by that time had achieved the status of a neurotransmitter in the brain, but there were other substances like serotonin, noradrenalin and dopamine, which could conceivably serve such a role and which had only recently been identified in the brain. Lysergic acid diethylamide, a drug that had attracted wide attention as an hallucinogen, had also been found to block some of the pharmacological actions of serotonin in the periphery. Three other psychotomimetic substances – mescaline, amphetamine and dimethyltryptamine – were recognised as congeners of serotonin or dopamine. About the same time, chlorpromazine had been found to be remarkably effective in the alleviation of psychotic behaviour and reserpine was being used extensively as a major tranquilliser. Knowledge of the remarkable ability of reserpine to deplete the brain of serotonin was being acquired in a laboratory of the National Heart Institute.

If the synapses involved in the mental states and behaviours produced or ameliorated by such drugs were chemically mediated, that would offer a plausible site at which these drugs could act. Moreover, if central synapses in general were chemical switches, then a biochemistry of behaviour was conceivable and, at the synapse, not only drugs but genetic factors, dietary constituents and hormones, metabolic, immune and infectious processes could all be seen to act, altering the patterns of trans-synaptic interaction and affecting behaviour and mental processes. For the first time, plausible and heuristic approaches could now be suggested and explored that might someday explain the biological disturbances in mental illness and the symptoms that depended upon them.

The most productive way of exploring these new approaches was not by way of a crash programme. The gap between the knowledge we had and the clinical problems was still too wide to be spanned by any concerted effort. What was needed was to narrow the gap by an increase in knowledge on both sides, which is best done by relying on the creativity and judgement of individual scientists who know better than anyone else what their next step should be. The members of the laboratory pursued their own research goals, some studying the clinical problems in greater detail and in the light of new knowledge, most expanding the base of fundamental knowledge in areas that they perceived to be relevant and feasible. Where appropriate, collaborative efforts developed within the laboratory and, quite as often, outside it.

Among the claims that were being made at that time was one postulating the formation of a toxic, hallucinogenic metabolite of circulating epinephrine in schizophrenia. It was difficult to evaluate that hypothesis because we knew little enough about the normal metabolism of epinephrine, let alone its metabolism in disease. By 1957, however, Julius Axelrod, one of the independent investigators in that laboratory, had discovered a major pathway in the catabolism of catecholamines and identified the major metabolites of epinephrine, and then turned his attention to norepinephrine and its inactivation at synapses in the periphery and in the brain. No support for an abnormal metabolism of catecholamines in schizophrenia has been adduced but the importance of catecholamines at central synapses is established, and their role in the action of several psychoactive drugs has been elucidated.

In 1961, after struggling with the decision for several months, I persuaded myself that it was not inappropriate for a biologist to serve as chairman of a department of psychiatry and accepted the Henry Phipps Professorship at Johns Hopkins. Believing as I did that the biological sciences were moving into psychiatry to enrich it and feeling that the search committee at Hopkins had taken a courageous step toward such a *rapprochement*, I could hardly decline. Despite a plea from a prominent psychoanalyst not to 'drive another nail into the coffin of psychiatry', but with the encouragement of Aubrey Lewis, whose breadth of understanding and far-sightedness I admired greatly, I assumed the post that Adolf Meyer had made famous. It was not long, however, before I realised that being chairman of a department of psychiatry and psychiatrist-in-chief of an important university hospital entailed more administrative responsibilities far beyond the field of research than I was comfortable with, and I resigned after a year with considerable regret.

Since my family had not moved from Bethesda, the long daily drives to Baltimore and back permitted me to think about and become committed to the prospect of carrying out a research strategy I had proposed two years earlier: a study of schizophrenia in adoptees and their two families as a means of dissociating the genetic and environmental variables. I could never have devoted the necessary time to such a project as chairman of a department of psychiatry, but my return to the NIMH was going to make it possible. There I found that David Rosenthal and Paul Wender had developed a similar commitment independently. We joined forces in a happy collaboration which has continued to this day. Our attempts to compile a total sample of adoptees in Maryland and the District of Columbia were not encouraging, but when we learned of the remarkable records which were maintained in Denmark and were able to elicit the invaluable collaboration of Fini Schulsinger, the plan became feasible and was eventually accomplished. The results of the studies which we have completed up until now support the operation of genetic factors in the etiology of a major segment of schizophrenic illness, in the affective disorders and in suicide. The adoption strategy also permits a search for the environmental influences which may be most important, and this has engaged our attention recently.

In circumstances prevailing in other branches of medicine, the demonstration of the chemical nature of synaptic transmission, the development of drugs capable of alleviating the symptoms of mental illness quite specifically and the elucidation of their synaptic actions, as well as the new evidence for genetic factors in the etiology of the major psychoses, would have ushered in an era of widespread public and professional support for the exploitation of the research opportunities that were then presented, but it was not to be as simple as that. The National Institute of Mental Health became dominated by quite a different philosophy in which research lost the high priority it had previously held, and biomedical research on schizophrenia was disparaged. Support of research requires a recognition of ignorance and the community psychiatry movement in the United States brooked no doubts regarding its convictions on the social etiology of mental illness and the types of social engineering required in order to treat and prevent it. The National Institute of Mental Health broke away from the National Institutes of Health. The Intramural Research Program, however, retained that affiliation and remained intact under the judicious and courageous leadership of

John Eberhart. The remainder of the NIMH was reorganised, in the course of which the Division of Extramural Research was fragmented and parochialised. Emphasis on research in the fundamental neurosciences was reduced on the premise that these had little relevance to psychiatry. At that point I decided to accept an invitation from Harvard to organise a biologically oriented programme in psychiatric research at the Massachusetts General Hospital and later at the McLean Hospital. Here, a consortium of scientists are working in fundamental and clinical research, ranging from neuroanatomy through genetics, molecular biology, pharmacology, psychology and pathology to clinical investigations. They, and their counterparts in several other departments of psychiatry, have been helping to strengthen the foundations of a more eclectic approach to the understanding, treatment and prevention of mental illness.

Current status of psychiatry

Psychiatry, if it is to fulfil the promises in its name, will recognise the manifold determinants of human behaviour and avoid simplistic approaches which claim to comprehend it in terms of a single theory or approach. It will accept the importance of the brain in mediating every movement and every mental state at the same time that it recognises the importance and irreducibility of the information and experience that it stores. The unique feature of the human brain is its ability to process, code and store experiential information and to utilise that store adaptively in later behaviour. Human behaviour is, to a considerable extent, determined by that experience, which, though mediated by biological mechanisms, cannot be reduced to them. The language we speak, the principles we value, the decisions that motivate our daily actions are to a greater extent a reflection of what we have learned than the result of how we were constituted. The differences among us in respect of these qualities are not to be found in the structure or chemical composition of our brains but lie largely within the scope of the psychological and social sciences.

It is useful to distinguish between the machinery that mediates behaviour and the stored information that is necessary to the evaluations and decisions which govern it. While the first of these determinants can effectively be investigated by the biological disciplines and modified by chemical intervention, the informational content and the system of values can be examined and influenced only by the disciplines and techniques that deal with the social and psychological context of experience. The oversimplifications of reductionism are readily refuted by any word in any language, whether in the form of the component letters or sounds or in the special perturbations in neuronal activity induced in the brain which perceives them. None of these symbols can tolerate much further reduction without loss of meaning. They can be explained and understood only in terms of the phenomenology and human experience that is condensed in them.

This inability to reduce informational content to structure, if not unique for the nervous system, is exaggerated by orders of magnitude there in comparison with the translational facility which appears to be attainable in genetics or immunology. The linkages between a gene, an enzyme and a function have been made comprehensible over the past few decades by the intellectual triumphs of molecular biology, as have the specificities of antigen–antibody complementarity. But in the case of the human brain, despite remarkable achievements in neurobiology, much of its behavioural output remains inexplicable in molecular terms. One need not invoke the transcendentalism of free will to account for the hiatus; sheer complexity offers a sufficient explanation.

It is not merely the number of neuronal units, variously estimated in the hundreds of billions, which creates this complexity, but the connections between them. Whereas the functions of muscle, liver or kidney may, to a large extent, be comprehended as a sum of the functions of their component units, the output of even a primitive brain depends predominantly upon the organisation of its components and the statistical properties of their activity. The role of each of these neurons depends upon its location, its connections, the present activity and the history of the network of which it is a part. The information storage, the comparisons and discriminations involved in a human decision are distributed over millions of neurons, making its description or comprehension at that level extremely remote.

But what of the severe disturbances of thought, behaviour and feeling that are seen in schizophrenia or in the heights and depths of manic-depressive illness? Are these merely the result of unusual rearing and interpersonal relationships, or adaptations to extremes of social stress, as some would have us believe? Or do they come about because of alterations in the biological mechanisms through which experience must operate?

It is futile any longer to argue that a particular mental disorder is biological or psychological in nature. The appropriate answers lie in the identification of the biological and the psychological components, evaluation of the contribution of each and, eventually, elucidation of the nature of the interactions among them. Although no responsible biochemist believes that his discipline is capable of distinguishing the brain of a Republican from that of a Democrat, he would have ample reason to feel that biochemical differences may exist in the case of the major mental illnesses: the characteristic features which can be mimicked by certain drugs or in the early stages of neurological or metabolic disease; the ability of other drugs specifically to ameliorate the symptoms by acting on synapses through which perception, cognition, affect and memory must occur; the chemical nature of the synapse which makes plausible the effects of chemical substances on behaviour and mental state; the evidence for important genetic contributions in the etiology of mental illness and the knowledge that the genes can express themselves only through biochemical processes.

Psychiatry, like the conditions it treats, is complex and heterogeneous in nature. There have been representatives of every point of view and the extreme positions, existing at the same time, have often contradicted each other. Even the anti-psychiatrists within psychiatry have promulgated conflicting dogmas: that mental illness is a myth, a creative adaptation to noxious social conditions or a range of diseases of the brain best treated by neurologists. The outstanding figures, however, and the most enduring positions have been those which recognised the heterogeneous nature of mental disorder, its multifactorial etiology and the different approaches which would be required for effective treatment and prevention. Henry Maudsley, more than 100 years ago, while emphasising the biological processes in mental illness, gave equal weight to the 'circumstances of life' and the 'behaviour of relatives and friends'. Sigmund Freud recognised that there were biological as well as experiential factors which, in themselves, were sometimes capable of producing mental illness and emphasised that it was the interaction between them which accounted for most. Eugen Bleuler invoked experiential and psychodynamic principles to describe the path from the morbid processes in the brain to the manifestations of mental illness. Adolf Meyer, who laid the groundwork for holistic and community psychiatry, continued his abiding interest in neuropathology and supported three distinguished laboratories of neurophysiology and experimental psychology at Johns Hopkins. Aubrey Lewis, while establishing a sound intellectual base for social psychiatry, never deviated from his recognition and support of the biological components of behaviour and mental illness.

If one discounts the temporary perturbations induced by vociferous extremists and views the most respected academic and research institutions of psychiatry as more representative of the field, one finds a basis for encouragement and optimism, if not complacency. Doctrinaire schools of thought, whether emphasising the exclusive importance of psychoanalytic, interpersonal, societal or orthomolecular approaches to mental disorder, are giving way to the more open-minded and eclectic position which recognises our large areas of ignorance regarding the etiology, pathogenesis, prevention and treatment of mental disorders and looks to research and the acquisition of new knowledge, rather than dogma, to lead the way. Within the field of research there is still some basis for concern, however. There is an overemphasis on premature demonstrations and costly evaluations of approaches to treatment and prevention without sufficient knowledge or evidence to justify the effort, at the cost of diminished support for fundamental research to elucidate the mysterious pathogenic processes which we are attempting to correct. There is criticism of the high cost of the imperfect approaches presently available for treatment but not the willingness to augment the inadequate fraction of that cost we allocate to the acquisition of knowledge. It is that, more than any other route, which will eventually lead to rational prevention as it has done repeatedly in the past.

The most competent and productive scientists are often motivated by the magnitude of a problem and the practical consequences of its solution, but they do not permit that to determine their research. They depend, instead, on a recognition of where their competence lies and the competence of the discipline they represent, the state of the art, the availability of new concepts, strategies and techniques, the originality and plausibility of the hypotheses they are able to generate and the feasibility of testing them. If psychiatric research were to be guided by the same principles, there would be a greater emphasis on fundamental research in the biological, behavioural and social sciences and less preoccupation with research that represents the premature application of inadequate knowledge and strategies to problems important enough to deserve better.

Future prospects of psychiatry

The phenomenal growth of knowledge in the neurosciences that has taken place in the past two decades would sustain a renewed search for the morbid processes in the brain which appear to underlie the major psychoses. There are new anatomical, molecular, biochemical and immunological techniques which constitute a new discipline of neuropathology which can be applied during life or *post mortem*. There can be little doubt that a further understanding of the chemical neurotransmitters that have been identified and others that remain to be characterised is an area of fundamental research which will ultimately be of considerable relevance. As neuropharmacologists learn more about the mechanism of action of the psychoactive drugs it should be possible to develop more specific agents with fewer side effects. Progress in all of these areas may be expected to lead to a more objective and explicit nosology and to permit the delineation of the modes of transmission and expression of genetic factors in those syndromes where they play a significant role.

The psychosocial milieu of the nuclear family represents an influence of obvious importance in acculturation and personality development; that influence can be further elucidated and its role in the genesis of the various types of mental illness more precisely evaluated. There are environmental factors other than psychological that may play a role in the etiology of mental disorders and these include perinatal factors, microbial and viral agents, dietary conditions and the manifold influences included under social stress which remain to be better defined.

If it appears that I have put too sharp a focus on mental illness and the medical model in this view of psychiatry, it is because I am very much of the opinion that psychiatry is a branch of medicine and that by training and tradition psychiatry is the only profession equipped to deal with mental illness in its various aspects. As for the medical model, that is merely the scientific method applied to illness. It need not be and has not, by tradition, been limited only to biology, but has involved the natural sciences, the behavioural sciences and the social sciences in its pursuit of the etiology, pathogenesis, diagnosis, treatment and prevention of illness. Human behaviour, of course, is considerably broader than that and the social and psychological sciences undoubtedly account for a larger share of the variance in human behaviour than does biology; but the entire field of human behaviour is not the domain of psychiatry.

Questions and answers

1. What training would you advocate for a would-be research worker in the field of biological psychiatry?

A good background in the neurosciences, psychology and psychiatry would be desirable. Since certification in each of these areas would require an unduly long period of training, familiarity with one or another of these fields may have to be acquired in an elective manner. In addition to the general training, concentration on at least one of the fundamental biological sciences would be essential, and one assumes a good knowledge of mathematics and statistics as a prerequisite. Since computers are being applied increasingly to problems in biological psychiatry and its cognate disciplines, facility in their use and knowledge of computer theory and programming would be desirable.

2. You state (page 92) that a 'responsible biochemist ... would have ample reason to feel that biochemical differences may exist in the case of the major mental illnesses'. Does this feeling extend to the so-called 'minor' illnesses (for example, the neuroses and personality disorders) and, if so, on what evidence?

The evidence for the assumption that biochemical disturbances occur in the pathogenesis of various mental diseases is most compelling for the major psychoses. In other disorders where psychosocial influences undoubtedly play a more important role, there is reason to believe that it need not be an exclusive one. There is evidence from adoption studies that severe alcoholism and sociopathy have a genetic component. There is more than 10 times the incidence of suicide in the biological relatives of adoptees who have committed suicide than in their adoptive relatives, and there have been several reports of biochemical changes in blood, cerebrospinal fluid and brain associated with an individual or family history of suicide. Comparable studies have not been carried out in the case of the neuroses, but one study found no increased concordance in monozygotic over dyzygotic twins for neuroses. There undoubtedly remain other forms of mental and behavioural deviance with and without diagnostic designations in which biological factors account for little if any of the variance.

3. In the light of the comment on human behaviour in your final sentence, how do you view the claims of behavioural medicine?

'Behavioural medicine' properly emphasises the role that psychological and social factors play, directly or indirectly, in the etiology, pathogenesis, treatment and prevention of medical and mental illness. Although the earlier claims that particular psychodynamic mechanisms operated in the etiology of specific somatic and mental disorders were not rigorously examined and have not been established, there is no doubt that psychological and emotional stressors effect visceral, endocrine and circulatory changes and that social and psychological factors produce deprivations or surfeits of important environmental ingredients and affect diet and lifestyles. Considerable compelling evidence exists that these influences can affect the course of most illnesses, initiate some and contribute favourably or unfavourably to the individual's adjustment to them.

Select bibliography

Kety, S. S. (1942). The lead citrate complexion and its role in the physiology and therapy of lead poisoning. *J. Biol. Chem.*, **142**, 181–92.

Kety, S. S., Woodford, R. B., Harmel, M. H., Freyham, F. A., Appel, K. E. & Schmidt, C. F. (1948). Cerebral blood flow and metabolism in schizophrenia. The effects of barbiturate semi-narcosis, insulin coma and electroshock. *Amer. J. Psychiat.*, **104**, 765–70.

Kety, S. S. & Schmidt, C. F. (1948). Nitrous oxide method for the quantitative determination of cerebral blood flow in man: theory, procedure and normal values. *J. Clin. Invest.*, **27**, 476–83.

Kety, S. S. (1950). Circulation and metabolism of the human brain in health and disease. *Amer. J. Med.*, **8**, 205–17.

Kety, S. S. (1951). The theory and applications of the exchange of inert gas at the lungs and tissues. *Pharmacol. Rev.*, **3**, 1–41.

Sokoloff, L., Wechsler, R. L., Mangold, R., Balls, K. & Kety, S. S. (1953). Cerebral blood flow and oxygen consumption in hyperthyroidism before and after treatment. *J. Clin. Invest.*, **32**, 202–8.

Mangold, R., Sokoloff, L., Conner, E., Kleinerman, J., Therman, P. G. & Kety, S. S. (1955). The effects of sleep and lack of sleep on the cerebral circulation and metabolism of normal young men. *J. Clin. Invest.*, **34**, 1092–100.

Kety, S. S. (1957). The general metabolism of the brain *in vivo*. In *Metabolism of the Nervous System*, ed. D. Richter, pp. 221–37. London: Pergamon Press.

Kety, S. S. (1959). Biochemical theories of schizophrenia. A two-part critical review of current theories and of the evidence used to support them. *Science*, **129**, 1528–32, 1590–6.

Kety, S. S. (1960). Measurement of local blood flow by the exchange of an inert, diffusible substance. In *Methods in Medical Research*, vol. VIII, ed. H. D. Brunner, pp.228–36. Chicago: Year Book Publishers.

Lewis, B. M., Sokoloff, L., Wechsler, R. L., Wentz, W. B. & Kety, S. S. (1960). A method for the continuous measurement of cerebral blood flow in man by means of radioactive krypton (Kr^{79}). *J. Clin. Invest.*, **39**, 707–16.

Kety, S. S. (1960). A biologist examines the mind and behavior. Many disciplines contribute to understanding human behavior, each with peculiar virtues and limitations. *Science*, **132**, 1861–70.

LaBrosse, E. H., Axelrod, J., Kopin, I. J. & Kety, S. S. (1961). Metabolism of $7H^3$epinephrine-d-bitartrate in normal young men. *J. Clin. Invest.*, **40**, 253–60.

Kety, S. S. (1961). The Academic Lecture: The heuristic aspects of psychiatry. *Amer. J. Psychiat.*, **118**, 385–97.

Kety, S. S., Rosenthal, D., Wender, P. H. & Schulsinger, F. (1968). The types and prevalence of mental illness in the biological and adoptive families of adopted schizophrenics. In *The Transmission of Schizophrenia*, ed. D. Rosenthal & S. S. Kety, pp. 345–62. Oxford: Pergamon Press.

Kety, S. S., Rosenthal, D., Wender, P. H., Schulsinger, F. & Jacobsen, B. (1975). Mental illness in the biological and adoptive families of adopted individuals who have become schizophrenic: a preliminary report based upon psychiatric interviews. In *Genetic Research in Psychiatry*, ed. R. Fieve, D. Rosenthal & H. Brill, pp. 147–165. Baltimore & London: The Johns Hopkins University Press.

Kety, S. S. (1974). From rationalization to reason. *Amer. J. Psychiat.*, **131**, 957–63.

Kety, S. S. (1978). The biological roots of mental illness: their ramifications through cerebral metabolism, synaptic activity, genetics and the environment. *Harvey Lectures Series 71*, pp. 1–22. New York: Academic Press.

Kety, S. S. (1978). Strategies of basic research. In: *Psychopharmacology: A Generation of Progress*, ed. M. A. Lipton, A. DiMascio & K. F. Killam, pp. 7–11. New York: Raven Press.

Kety, S. S. (1980). The 52nd Maudsley Lecture. The syndrome of schizophrenia: unresolved problems and opportunities for research. *Br. J. Psych.*, **136**, 421–36.

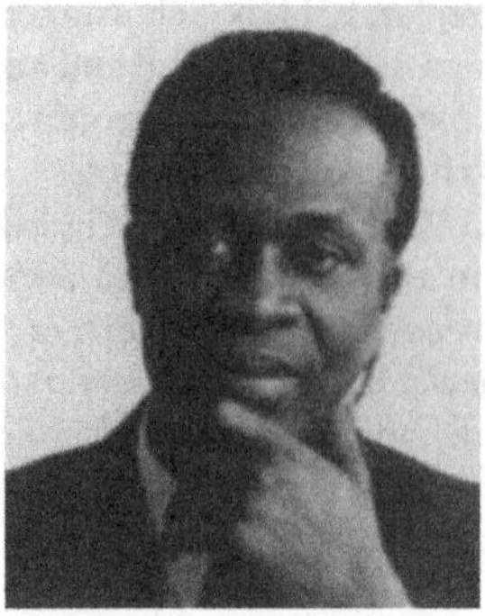

7 · THOMAS LAMBO

Personal background and professional experience

I was born in Abeoukuta, Nigeria, on 29 March 1923. I obtained my medical degrees at the University of Birmingham in 1948 and hold postgraduate degrees in psychological medicine and psychiatry.

After holding senior posts at the General Hospital and the Midland Nerve Hospital in Birmingham, I served in Nigeria where in 1960 I became a senior specialist at the Neuropsychiatric Centre of the Western Region Ministry of Health. During these years I became convinced that any effective efforts towards better mental health must rest upon precise knowledge of the society concerned, and this led to my pioneering work on the psychosocial aspects of mental disorders in Africa. One aspect of this work was the development of an experimental community mental health scheme at Aro, later filmed by the United Nations in *The Healers of Aro*.

In 1963 I became Professor of Psychiatry and Head of the Department of Psychiatry, Neurology and Neurosurgery at the University of Ibadan. While continuing to hold this chair, I was made Dean of the Medical School at the University of Ibadan in 1966 and Vice-Chancellor in 1968.

In 1971 I joined the World Health Organisation (WHO)as Assistant Director-General with special responsibility for the Divisions of Mental Health, Non-communicable Diseases, Therapeutic and Prophylactic Substances and Health Manpower Development. I was appointed the

Deputy Director-General of the Organisation in 1973. I am a member of the Club of Rome and became the first African member of the Vatican's Pontifical Academy of Sciences in 1974.

During my career I have published more than 150 articles and I have also written a number of monographs; my monograph *Psychiatric Disorders among the Yorubas* was published in 1963. My more recent publications reflect my current interest in a variety of subjects, including the responsibility of science in developing countries, the humanisation of consciousness, the role of the central nervous system in the attainment of the quality of life, and cultural and social aspects of child care in developing countries.

I am married and have three sons.

Current status of psychiatry

> I have examined the brain and found
> no trace of love.
>
> *J. W. Rowntree, 1949*

Since the data of experience have proved that a materialistic and mechanistic view of man and his needs and aspirations, his happiness and total well-being are grossly inadequate, a multi-dimensional view of man has emerged in which one finds the various disciplines complementing and bringing new knowledge, rather than contradicting each other. In attempting to solve the health problems of individuals and nations with diverse socio-cultural backgrounds, in promoting global social and human development, in understanding man and his behaviour, in our effort to bring about the transformation of some of the basic human values – dignity, equity, liberty, security, free choice – into manageable health objectives, it is inconceivable to think that we can acquire new knowledge of man without interaction and integration with many disciplines.

It is with relief that one turns to great thinkers like Heisenberg (1952) who recognised that 'the concepts "soul" and "life" do not occur in atomic physics', or to Gilbert Ryle (1949) who asserted that 'the mind of man is not a matter interpreted by the quantum theory'. According to them, human existence shows other kinds of forms which we cannot match with mathematical forms of modern physics. If we want to describe mental or living processes (human development, human behaviour, social relations, values, promotion of total human well-being, etc.) we have to introduce yet other concepts. These concepts have been and are being provided by the roles which psychiatry and the social sciences are vigorously playing in international health.

Health, in its broad concept, and as an integral part of global social and human development (socio-economic) strategy, has assumed an extraordinarily complex, multifaceted status over the last two decades. This importance has been due not, as one would like to think, to the recent great advances and unprecedented revolution in biology and medicine but to pressing social, human and economic factors. The frightening truth is that the problems of all contemporary societies are themselves compounded by political, economic, social, psychological and technological elements. The multi-variant components of the *problématique* can hardly be correctly and realistically formulated, let alone solved, by the politician in isolation, by the economist, the molecular biologist, the health administrator, the clinician, the engineer, the sociologist or the psychiatrist. These problems constitute a phenomenon of a kind for which it seems impossible to see how any explanation in terms of observable phenomena could ever be adequately provided.

The World Health Organisation, which ushered in a new era of international health in 1948 and which defines health as 'a state of complete physical, mental and social well-being and not merely the absence of disease or infirmity', has discovered a number of frightening facts. These include the perennial prescriptions by the United Nations of universal panaceas over succeeding development decades; man's continued deterioration, lack of social justice in health, insensitivities of the nations that possess formidable arsenals of scientific knowledge, resources and manpower; a deepening conflict between nations and the sense of separation; and a state of deprivation, which Hegel calls alienation. Søren Kierkegaard would certainly have regarded the whole situation as essentially a tragedy of the human state.

The developing world itself has profound feelings of desertion, of isolation from hope, knowledge and being. WHO has discovered this to be a perception of man's condition, hidden from the complacent and self-satisfied bureaucrats and obvious to every sensitive spirit. However, like Arthur Koestler, WHO sees the polarisation between the affluent North and the deprived South, between the rich and the poor as 'the laughing few and the screaming multitude'.

It is now over 35 years since the signing of the United Nations Charter which inaugurated an international effort to establish a new international order. This constituted one of the most striking and hopeful features of the UN. Among many obscure pronouncements on humanitarian ideals and the kinship of men were some concrete instruments aimed at achieving greater human ends or meeting human aspirations; they sought to guarantee security and needs in a new human context, and to formulate a policy by the great 'civilised' governments to extirpate social and economic slavery from the world and release human energy and potentialities in the way William James defined them. These aims were thought to be right. What is right, however, need not necessarily be true.

Today, that international order has reached a critical turning point; its hopes of creating a better life for the whole human family, and of transforming society, have turned out to be illusory. It has proved impossible to meet the minimum health and social needs. On the contrary, more people are now hungry, sick, homeless and illiterate than when the UN was first set up to erase all these inequalities and the dearth of opportunities. These and others are phenomena which appear only on the psychological level, and accordingly, science must first approach them on this level, as Julian Huxley and C. H. Waddington once pointed out in their discussion of values.

To these preoccupations must be added the realisation that the next three decades may bring a doubling of the world population. Another world on top of this one, equal in numbers, demands and hopes.

The problem today is not primarily one of absolute physical shortage but of economic and social maldistribution and misuse; mankind's predicament is rooted primarily in economic, intellectual, social and political structures, and in behaviour within and between countries.

Millions of people die prematurely because of a failure to put scientific knowledge to work through strong government and public health programmes. We suffer because the public health programmes are not as strong as their knowledge and techniques; we suffer from a shortage of appropriate techniques for the prevention and control of many diseases; we suffer equally from a shortage of knowledge regarding the circumstances which follow the development of psychiatric disorders as much as we suffer from the defiant arrogance of Western culture which sets up its civilisation as the standard by which all the other civilisations are to be measured. We suffer because of the perpetuation of rigid patterns and stratification of health care systems, and we suffer because of a lack of economic resources to translate scientific knowledge into action.

In formulating strategies for international health with emphasis on global social and human development, several questions often recur. What are the conditions under which real communication can be developed between people of different cultures, with different life experiences and different value systems, so that each nation or group can help others to new appreciation, for example WHO's programme of technical co-operation? What points of entry to co-operation between nations of different ideologies and social systems can one find through human problems which they have in common, such as mental illness, psychosocial factors in health, crime and delinquency, alcoholism, drug dependence and guidance within schools? It is for such reasons that our efforts and many of our activities, including those in the research area, are directed towards the application of what our experience has shown to be the most effective measure in meeting the global health problems, namely the provision of primary health care.

The essence of primary health care is described in detail in several WHO publications:

> Primary health care addresses the main health problems in the community, providing promotive, preventive, curative and rehabilitation services accordingly. Since these services reflect and evolve from the economic conditions and social values of the country and its communities, they will vary by country and community, but will include at least: promotion of proper nutrition and an adequate supply of safe water; basic sanitation; maternal and child care, including family planning; immunization against the major infectious diseases; prevention and control of locally endemic diseases; education concerning prevailing health problems and the methods of preventing and controlling them; and appropriate treatment for common diseases and injuries.
>
> Primary health care is likely to be most effective if it employs means that are understood and accepted by the community and applied by community health workers at a cost the community and the country can afford. These community health workers, including traditional practitioners, where applicable, will function best if they reside in the community they serve and are properly trained socially and technically to respond to its expressed health needs.

I have dwelt on these important aspects of international health, of global social and human development to emphasise the complexity of the problems which lie on the frontiers of psychiatry and the social sciences. They also stress the enlarged obligations and roles of psychiatry, especially when dealing with the relative importance of such factors as national status, temperament, economic and social conditions, group connections, national loyalties and value systems, situational pressures and other immediate motivations in predicting individual and national capacity to accept technical co-operation and make constructive use of new ideas.

We can see at a glance now that almost everything of interest to man, especially everything that impinges upon his social life, lies beyond a physico-chemical explanation. This is the main reason why many years ago WHO insisted on the use of the term 'mental health'. At the same time WHO recognises the need for using the insights of the social sciences and psychiatry in the formulation of global social and health objectives; in dealing with health problems; in initiating the process of social transformation; in resolving conflicts and promoting the ideology of national self-reliance, and in enhancing the ability of the countries to maintain themselves as resilient and growing organisms with abundant desire and capacity for change and choice-making. WHO also accepts the need to relate programmes in specific areas to one another and to the larger problems of social and human development, thereby preventing the development of vertical programmes. In addition, WHO realises that the relationship between different nations should be one of mutual respect and responsibility, and that technical co-operation between them in the field of health should be fostered by recognition of common problem areas in which work might be carried out concurrently. With proper motivation and effective utilisation of their human resources, even the least developed of the developing countries can enhance their quality of life.

The need to use all the insights of mental health and increase the role of psychiatry became critical when WHO decided to line up squarely and unequivocally with the unprotected, deprived and exploited nations. Here there was not only a rejection of mere materialism but also an insistence on the priority of the quality of life, of love and of hope, when WHO came out with exciting but relevant programmes embracing all sectors of development, needing the full participation of all countries, especially the need to transfer appropriate technology and scientific techniques from the developed to the developing countries.

To undertake this task, psychiatry within the context of international health has had not only to assume some of its traditional roles with more refined and reliable scientific tools and techniques, such as the treatment of mental illness, the treatment of the sick and the deviant, and their rehabilitation, but also to accept new responsibilities. These include the promotion of mental health, the mental health implications of rapid social change which tend to produce ambiguity and conflict between traditional values on the one hand and new norms on the other, the analysis of psychosocial factors in health, the social and behavioural aspects of health, the study and analysis of the meaning of the quality of life in different social and cultural contexts, and the determination and evaluation of mental health needs and resources within communities.

This assumption of new roles can be accomplished only by close collaboration with social and behavioural disciplines and close co-operation with statesmen, policy-makers, health administrators, scientists and others in positions of responsibility. This approach to the promotion of social, human and cultural growth requires a degree of knowledge of group dynamics of a specialised kind. The insights and skills which psychiatry and allied social sciences have made available must be utilised extensively in spite of the obvious shortcomings in their techniques and methodologies. They can enable individuals, especially those in power within the nation to discover for themselves ways of improving the patterns of human relations and social adjustments, and at the same time may awaken an urgent sense of need to change the habits of their daily thinking and behaviour. The process can also lead to a total mobilisation of human and community resources to participate in all activities that will enhance their growth and development.

Without such a fundamental change in the attitude and type of working relationship it is extremely doubtful whether any changes of a lasting nature will occur in the field of international health and development – social and human – at a global level, however desirable they may be or however clearly the justification for such changes may have been explained to all concerned. It is therefore obvious that the sound effective approach to international health as an integral part of total development is psycho-cultural and multiprofessional. The overriding technique used is '*open-ended*', belonging to the projective category.

What possibilities exist to institute early warning and monitoring systems; to develop social indicators, sensitive and sophisticated enough to identify individuals and families in distress; to ameliorate adverse social and material conditions and enhance the quality of life for those at the bottom of the social and economic pyramid; and to identify such special high-risk groups as migrants, refugees, minorities and people in transition? Value systems will continue to undergo enormous change and family roles will, of necessity, be modified. If man and his family are to remain syntonic with the emerging necessities in a developing milieu, the adequate design of multidisciplinary tools from several disciplines will have to be made to assist in this task. The role of psychiatry in this task is indispensable, if not imperative.

Although science and technology in the health sciences have provided some remarkable tools, especially within the last two decades, these major advances in the knowledge and application of high-level technology have, in some ways, become great obstacles to this much-needed change in the right direction. The threat of technological neo-colonialism is real, leading to many factors which impede true and relevant development. For example, there is the domination of human life by technology; an over-emphasis on urban-centred curative care to the detriment, and at the expense, of preventive and rehabilitative services, especially in the developing countries; the soaring expenditures in health services; and the cost of health care which only the most affluent minority can afford.

These advances in science and technology have not yet fully helped us to promote the concrete and valuable economic and social development which is of basic importance to the fullest attainment of health for all in our contemporary society and to the reduction of the gap between the health status of the small group of *élite* and the underprivileged masses, between the urban population and the rural, giving priority to those most in need, especially the vulnerable groups, such as migrants, workers, students, children and the disabled. Since these groups are normally faced with many adverse psycho-social factors it is a matter of urgency to guarantee a level of health which will permit every citizen of this country to lead a socially and economically productive life.

For these and other reasons WHO, while encouraging the development of science and technology in health, has had to politicise health issues so as to mobilise strong political, intellectual and moral forces in a positive way, that is bring about a *health revolution*, in the developing countries where those crippling traditions have not yet established themselves into formidable obstacles. The politics of health is rough because of the vested interest of the profession, with its built-in ultra-conservatism; the Ministries of Health in many countries have little political visibility and weight within their national cabinets. The rating of national priority puts health much lower down the scale; traditionally, there is also a tendency not to associate health with or relate it to other sectors of development.

The magnitude and complexity of this task corresponds to the importance of its achievement for the troubled and insecure world of today. The full attainment of the goals described in the subsequent section of this chapter requires not only a clear understanding of the values currently missing in our cultures, together with an appreciation of the strengths and potentials which do exist, but a similar appreciation and awareness of the inadequacies, actual and latent, in the methods used to approach problems of development by the representatives of other nations.

Many of the problems associated with, or inherent in, international health, especially in global social and human development, lie beyond the scope of orthodox medicine, including psychiatry, and must always remain outside the purview of 'medicine' in its classical sense. Our image of social reality and human experience is today more unsettled and uncertain than it has been for a long time, especially now that we confronted with the fragmentation of science into highly specialised, isolated branches, and with its use as an instrument of irresponsible power.

We must aim at a new professional and scientific ecumenicalism in spite of the differences inherent in our approach, technique and methods and concepts, and must cultivate genuine consultative and interdisciplinary intercourse. We know that some of these concepts, especially those dealing with the nature of man, will profit from being merged into one. Our mind must seek unity.

Psychiatry and the developing world

One of the most devastating forms of illness in the developing countries today is the group of communicable diseases. Malaria, the acute diarrhoeal diseases, respiratory infections, childhood infections, tuberculosis, preventable blindness, toxoplasmosis, cerebrospinal meningitis, smallpox and encephalomyelitis, trypanosomiasis, soil-transmitted helminthiasis and other endemic and epidemic diseases continue to contribute heavily to an intolerably high level of mortality and morbidity and to an impaired quality of life in most developing countries.

South American trypanosomiasis is endemic in Argentina, Venezuela and Brazil. Tsetse-borne trypanosomiasis, sleeping sickness, in some 10 million square kilometres of tropical Africa is a most formidable obstacle to the development of the continent and remains one of the important pathogenic agents in some types of chronic brain syndrome. Endemic goitre accounts for a sizeable population of mentally subnormal people in some of the developing countries, for example Ecuador, where a survey of school children in 1957 showed that endemic goitre was a serious public health problem. The incidence varied from 30 per cent to 67 per cent in the Andean provinces. The effects included mental retardation, deaf-mutism and endemic cretinism.

To all these can be added malnutrition, alcoholism, drug abuse, cardiovascular disease, major psychiatric disorders, cancer and other non-communicable diseases whose incidence and prevalence are rising steeply. Apart from this, it has now been shown that in the developing countries up to one-fifth of all the contacts of general health care services are with people whose problems are largely, if not mainly, psychological.

The major psychiatric diseases in developing countries are those commonly found elsewhere, for example the schizophrenias, depressive disorders and neuroses, but the natural histories of these disorders vary a great deal from those occurring in the industrialised societies. Between these clinical entities there are numerous gradations engendered by peculiarities of culture, social forces and/or genetic factors, such as some atypical exotic syndromes (Lambo, 1962; Yap, 1951).

In most of these countries there is a reportedly high prevalence of epilepsy and convulsive disorders. Many cases of epilepsy in Africa are known to be due to trauma, poor obstetric care, poor maternal and child care, birth injury and neonatal infection. Epilepsy and convulsive disorders are widely distributed in the developing countries of Africa, Asia and Latin America. In tropical Africa Piraux found that 30 per cent of epileptic patients had real and intractable social problems. In the mountains of Venezuela 40 per cent of the patients attending a psychiatric clinic were epileptic, some with schizophrenic-like psychoses and some with depression.

In my review of psychiatry in the tropics, I concluded: 'Massive preventive programmes against nutritional deficiencies, and infections and other endemic diseases, would reduce psychiatric morbidity by well over 40 per cent' (Lambo, 1965). This observation remains true up until today and carries implications for health services, especially social and preventive medicine. My own prediction for psychiatry was a new and demanding role (Lambo, 1956); in view of the unique and varied nature of the social and health problems facing it, psychiatry will have to lose its traditional and self-imposed isolation and privacy.

The development of modern psychiatric services has been slow in the developing countries and even in some of the developed countries. When and where these have been developed, they have been separated from the main stream of the general health services. Most of the developing countries have inherited the prejudice against psychiatry which prevailed in the countries of the old colonial powers and have underrated the priority for psychiatry services. Most of the resistance to the development of proper psychiatric services was met within the medical profession and this also accounted for the delay in instituting training centres and psychiatric departments in the medical schools.

Today the profile is different, not simply because psychiatry has re-orientated itself from its orthodox and historical past, but also because it has assumed the wider responsibilities thrust upon it by the demands of society and health. In its attempt at adaptation to new needs and demands, psychiatry has had to develop more sensitive scientific techniques and methodologies, especially for the prevention and control of diseases. It has strengthened its link with medicine as an important branch without losing its *artistry*, and some of its essential methods deal with human processes which cannot be subjected to rigorous mathematical measurements and which remain resistant to evaluation and inaccessible to scientific techniques and logical analysis. This must remain a part of psychiatry's identity.

In Sir Aubrey Lewis' words (1958): 'This is not to deny the large part which compassion and human feeling must play in the care of mental disorder ... its history attests that they will always be necessary; but they operate in a territory that must be explored and chartered ....' Even the new biology which ushered in a scientific revolution still reproaches the mechanistic way of thinking with its failure to understand wholeness in the process of life.

In many of the developing countries psychiatry has blazed new trails and introduced a number of dynamic innovations in the field of therapeutic modalities. These include village systems, mobile mental health teams, psychiatric sections in general hospitals and various types of community psychiatry, coupled with the mobilisation of the community, especially the family, collaboration with indigenous health and medical practitioners. Some traditional healers have proved to be great exponents of the affective aspects of ritual participation and some remain supreme in dealing with the dynamic interrelatedness of symbolic phenomena and socio-cultural organisation, proving themselves adept in promoting critical thresholds of group effectiveness. The training of various cadres of mental health workers has featured prominently in many national health plans.

As I see it, psychiatry, especially in the developing countries, is moving in the direction of progress, dictated by needs. This change has been brought about by what I may call 'moral experience' to borrow Bertrand Russell's phrase. Psychiatric practice no longer unconsciously exhibits any symptom of 'the flight from science' (*Br. Med. J.* 1980). Good, solid clinical observation, uncontaminated by emotion and empiricism of the West or by any *a priori* commitment to any school of thought, is bringing forward new insights into general psychopathology, especially in the realm of the neuroses. Psychiatry in the developing countries has gained intellectual and academic weight and commands political visibility equal to that of any important branch of medicine.

This intellectual respectability is partly due to the fact that the psychiatrist in the developing country has effectively and primarily played the role of a 'doctor' and is seen and regarded as a physician. He also strives to understand the wholeness of life. In this task the psychiatrist in the developing countries, faced with social, cultural and psychological dimensions of health of a different order, will find that the old method of arrangement of clinical facts into consistent chains of inference to formulate a hypothesis, followed by the use of data to test and occasionally to refine the hypothesis, is still a rewarding method of clinical investigation.

In view of the rapid social change taking place in the developing countries, the rapid and convulsive acculturation, the contradictory values, rapid urbanisation and uprooting, coupled with psychosocial factors, alienation and confusion of identity, there is much to be gained in the practice of psychiatry by the provision of an empirical framework necessary for generalisation which may differ in many ways from the theories based on clinical material from the West. The developing countries represent a unique social and human laboratory and a vast area of the 'universe' for renewed scientific consideration to which one might apply Sir Francis Bacon's comment, 'that many excellent and useful matters are yet laid up in the bosom of Nature... quite out of the common of our imagination, and still undiscovered; but they too will doubtless be brought to light in the course and revolution of years'.

Clinical psychiatrists and psychologists practising in the developing countries could, with advantage, decontaminate themselves intellectually from Freudian and neo-Freudian theories and advance new clinical insights and new knowledge in the unwieldy area of comparative psychopathology. Freud's theories and those of his disciples nonetheless represent, at their best, a spectrum of possible ideas emanating from Hellenic and Judaeo-Christian culture and tradition. Psychoanalysis has been a potent instrument of research and for testing theories. Heuristically it retains its importance for this reason.

Psychiatry and science

It is easy to regard the early approach or the introduction to the problem of psychiatry and science as a form of systems philosophy of human values or even as a dialectical aspect of social and moral development. There is, in fact, no dichotomy between facts and values. The entirely medical view of the role of psychiatry is wrong, not in what it asserts or contributes but in what it omits. Goethe's rebuke of Newton is often quoted in this connection, mainly because Newton, in order to carry out his experiment on the nature of light, first shut himself in a dark room, the window of which had but a small open slit, and then investigated the light that had been mistreated: 'And truly, how little is left in this experiment of the living light around us.'

Within WHO psychiatry has embraced and encouraged the rigorous methods of scientific enquiry in all WHO collaborating centres by extending its power beyond nature, a process of experimental method in the service of knowledge. It has encouraged the development of the methods of the natural sciences – biochemistry and physiology – and the social and behavioural sciences, as well as sound clinical methods. No one would pick a quarrel with Rothman's (1962) warning when he writes '... unless our philosophy of science becomes more critical, experimental, more deductive and inventive, we will remain in the Renaissance period of medical history, awaiting a Harvey to catapult us into the seventeenth century ...'.

In the sphere of international health psychiatry has had to collaborate with the programmes of many medical specialities, especially in the realm of the prevention and control of diseases. Such collaboration has involved programmes of maternal and child health, of human reproduction, of the strengthening of health services and of medical education. Its own programmes have included the scientific study of the major psychiatric disorders (epidemiology, prevention and control); community and social psychiatry, including manpower development; studies of common neurological disorders; prevention and treatment of drug dependence; alcohol-related problems; biological psychiatry and psychopharmacology; mental health legislation; psychosocial aspects of health; and biomedical and health services research.

At this juncture it would seem appropriate to describe very briefly some of the important research that psychiatry has initiated at the global level and which, in my view, has bestowed on the subject a pre-eminent position and has persuaded policy-makers, scientific colleagues and health administrators to take the discipline seriously. Here it is important to refer to those who have moulded the subject in this way. Great tribute must be paid to Dr Norman Sartorius, the Director of the Division of Mental Health, WHO, and his team who, over the years, have imbued this subject with strict scientific rigour and discipline. This move was preceded by a drastic overhaul and reformulation of the programme through 'a process of consultation within WHO, with other UN bodies, with governments, the world scientific community and the non-governmental organisations in psychiatry, mental health, social and behavioural sciences' (WHO, 1978*a*).

I will attempt to summarise the research strategies of WHO's mental health programme, which has emphasised the role of psychiatry, giving an outline of research activities that are being initiated, co-ordinated and supported by the programme at country, regional and global level. Research activities within the programme are geared primarily towards providing knowledge which would help to achieve the following objectives:

(i) to prevent or reduce psychiatric, neurological and psychosocial problems, including those related to alcohol and drug dependence;

(ii) to increase the effectiveness of general health services through appropriate utilization of mental health skills and knowledge;

(iii) to develop strategies for intervention based on an increased awareness of the mental health aspects of social action and change.

The research component of the programme (Sartorius, 1980*b*) also aims to serve other important purposes of WHO: to help orientate attention of research workers to prevalent and socially relevant problems; to strengthen local research potential, particularly in the developing countries; to generate appropriate research methods, instruments and other tools, and ensure that training in their use is widely available; and to facilitate the establishment of equitable collaboration between countries in matters of research. All WHO research is carried out in collaboration with institutions and individuals in member countries of WHO. Funds come from the WHO budget, from the participating institutions and, on occasion, from governmental and non-governmental agencies which support research.

Future prospects of psychiatry

Research themes

1. The development of a common language

An essential prerequisite for collaboration in the field of mental health is agreement on a language which can be understood and will be used by all concerned. Such an agreement must cover terms used in the description of mental and neurological functioning and pathology (including diagnosis); indicators of mental, neurological and psycho-social problems, for example those related to alcohol and drug dependence, and of the success of measures undertaken for their solution; terms referring to environmental factors or situations relevant to mental health investigations; and methods of investigations, for example how biological samples are obtained and sent to other centres.

Instruments for the assessment of specific conditions have also been developed. Thus, for example, an instrument for the assessment of depressive disorder has resulted from a multi-national study of depression (Sartorius, 1975). This instrument has now been tested in nine countries and exists in Bulgarian, Danish, English, French, German, Hindi, Japanese, Persian and Polish versions. It covers the clinical state, psychiatric history and socio-demographic data and was found to be applicable and acceptable in the populations studied (Sartorius *et al.* 1980; Jablensky *et al.*, 1981). Instruments for the assessment of alcohol- and drug-related problems are being developed in the framework of the projects on community response to alcohol-related problems and in the research and reporting programme on drug dependence, to be described later.

In the WHO study concerned with psychosomatic changes occurring in women after tubal ligation, instruments for the assessment of reproductive life and history were developed, drawing on experience obtained in previous studies and adding parts needed for the study. This strategy has also been used in developing a series of other instruments. The first drafts of assessment instruments usually contain modules tested in the context of other schedules in a variety of cultures. As a result, the development lag in studies for which new instruments are needed can be substantially shortened.

Instruments for the assessment of impairments, handicaps and associated disabilities in psychiatric patients are being tested in eight countries in Europe and in the Sudan. Disability in patients with schizophrenic disorders is being assessed first, before extending the work to other groups of patients suffering from mental and physical disorders.

2. *Characteristics of mental and neurological disorders and of psychosocial problems of major public health importance*

(a) Schizophrenic syndromes. WHO's first major research effort was concerned with schizophrenia. The International Pilot Study of Schizophrenia (WHO, 1973) was launched to establish whether it is feasible to carry out collaborative projects in psychiatry according to a commonly agreed protocol and with the active involvement of investigators from

different countries. Centres in Denmark, Columbia, China, India, Nigeria, Czechoslovakia, the United Kingdom, United States and USSR participated in a study in which series of patients consecutively admitted to psychiatric facilities were examined by means of standardised research instruments. The study proved that international collaboration in psychiatric research is feasible. It also produced instruments for the standardised assessment of patients in different cultures and contributed to our knowledge about schizophrenia by demonstrating that: (i) similar schizophrenic syndromes exist in all of the cultural settings included in the study; but that (ii) the course and outcome of schizophrenia show significant differences between countries, patients in developing countries having on the whole a more favourable course and outcome than their counterparts in the developed world (WHO, 1979).

(b) Acute psychoses. Acute psychoses, often described as the most frequent reason for admission to hospitals in developing countries, are being investigated in Ibadan, Agra, Chandigarh, Cali and Aarhus to obtain information which will lead to a better psychopathological delineation of the syndrome and facilitate further sociological, clinical and biological studies. Methods developed in the study of determinants of outcome of severe mental disorders and in other WHO projects will be used in this investigation, with appropriate additions now being developed on the basis of an analysis of case-histories of patients with acute psychoses seen in the centres collaborating in the study and elsewhere, for example Algeria.

(c) Alcohol-related problems. The growing realisation that alcohol-dependence syndromes represent only a part of alcohol-related problems, ranging from cirrhosis to traffic accidents, as well as recent developments pointing the way to effective intervention in the field, has revived WHO's commitment to action in this field. After surveys of the situation in various countries a major research project has been initiated to explore the response of communities to alcohol-related problems.

(d) Depressive disorders. A programme of investigation on depressive disorders was started in 1972. This programme contains studies with an epidemiological orientation, biological studies and operational research (Sartorius, 1975, 1980*a*; Sartorius & Jablensky, 1981).

(e) Drug dependence. Evaluative research is an important component of

all projects dealing with the implementation of programmes designed to reduce the demand for dependence-producing drugs.

(f) Neurological disorders. A programme concerned with the control of neurological disorders was started in the early 1970s. It involves leading neuroscience centres in Canada, France, Mexico, Nigeria, Senegal, Switzerland, the United States and USSR (Bolis, 1978*a*, *b*). The centres are engaged in several WHO-coordinated research activities, including a study of markers for the differential diagnosis of epilepsy being carried out in Bethesda, Ibadan, Marseilles, Mexico and Montreal, and utilising the exceptional diagnostic facilities existing in these centres. The same centres, as well as the centre in Moscow, are also engaged in a study of transient ischaemic cerebrovascular attacks.

3. The development and improvement of treatment methods

A new set of studies dealing with the effectiveness of medicaments has been undertaken recently. The largest of these is the WHO coordinated study of the effects of psychotropic drugs in different populations (WHO, 1978*b*).

4. The organisation of mental health services: assessment and development of new models

A major aim of WHO's co-operation with countries is the improvement of provision of mental health care. To ensure that appropriate advice is provided to governments wishing to improve mental health care, several studies have been initiated.

5. The psychosocial aspects of general health care and high-risk group research

One of the principal mental health programme objectives deals with the application of mental health knowledge to general health care provision.

It is my aim and belief that an interchange of opinion and knowledge from differing standpoints and disciplines should be freely and aggressively prosecuted in all that pertains to the optimal development of man. The mental horizon and the quality and effectiveness of the skills of psychiatrists and of those of other workers whose circles of activities impinge on our own will then be materially widened, to the enduring advantage of the individual and society alike.

Questions and answers

1. In the light of your argument, how do you account for the emergence of the anti-psychiatry movement in recent years?

Since the anti-psychiatry movement is not a new phenomenon, I would rather speak of its re-emergence in recent years.

In my opinion, this has not been due to one single factor but to a combination of many factors, social, economic, religious and cultural. Because of psychiatry's isolation from the mainstream of general medicine, and because, in a way, it is allied with philosophy, religion and those disciplines which tend to depend on subjective evaluation, it has always been both hated and loved: hated, because man possesses many crude, primitive, unconscious motivations which he tries to conceal – any discipline that tries to unravel these primitive traits is bound to be unpopular – and loved, because it touches upon existential concerns of central significance.

Psychiatry has too often been equated with psychoanalysis, a subject which, over the years, has earned itself a reputation that is not entirely satisfactory, either scientifically or socially.

Psychiatric advances have been very slow and research in psychiatry has been disappointingly slow in its progress. It has been said by many influential people, especially in the developing countries, that intelligent young doctors striving towards a prestigious professional career should enter specialities such as surgery, gynaecology, neurosurgery or internal medicine, and those physicians who go into psychiatry have often been regarded as being either intellectually inferior or inexplicably eccentric.

In this connection I would like to refer to the comment which I made in 1975:

> I believe that it should be possible for psychiatry to survive its present moral crisis and become a positive instrument for the promotion of health, security, and freedom of individuals, to free men from servitude (to nature, to ignorance and disease, to other men, to institutions, to beliefs) considered oppressive. The aim here is to release men from the bondage of these servitudes and/or to enhance their opportunities for self-actualization, however conceived, and, finally, to assist in the formulation of the perceptions of our total human situation.
>
> Pinel, Chiarugi and Tuke were the standard bearers of the courageous and epoch-making movements which dissociated psychiatry from an outmoded set of beliefs, habits and social and

medical institutions. In spite of their differences, they had this major ethical and moral principle in common, 'that they did not sit in moral judgement on the patients, nor treat outrageous and dissolute conduct as a culpable fall from grace'.

Can we as psychiatrists and men and women of unalloyed intellectual and scientific integrity be committed to certain ethical responsibility and moral principles, develop greater sensitivity and consciousness for critical social and political issues, and unhesitatingly subscribe to the doctrine 'That man is the highest being for man; to the categorical imperative to overthrow all conditions in which man is humiliated, enslaved, despised and rejected being'? Psychiatry itself is not the real danger, for psychiatry will not hurt human freedom unless men direct it to such ends. This means that the problem centres not on scientific technology, but on moral philosophy and the social scientific disciplines.

Because the theory and practice of psychiatry are not neutral to human and social existential concerns, all these factors make it an all too easy target for a kind of 'paranoid projection', as my psychodynamically minded colleagues might say. In a way, it is convenient to blame a rather heterogeneous and not too coherent professional group for the society's ills.

In these brief remarks on the anti-psychiatry movement I have not dealt with some other cultural and social factors tending to alienate the psychiatric patient from his family and society, which cause shame to be cast on the family, nor with the historical and traditional association of the concept of insanity across cultures.

2. You refer to the need to 'politicise health issues'. How do you apply this need to the field of psychiatry?

There is no doubt in my mind that in order to bring about a health revolution within psychiatry we have to overcome many obstacles, some of which are inherent in the profession itself. For example, in developing countries not only are the available financial and manpower resources inadequate; their meagre resources are mainly used to cater for a small percentage of the population (the *élite* group). This is equally true of psychiatric care in many of the developed countries.

With regard to general medicine and health services, the most formidable obstacle has been said to be the technicalisation of health. This phenomenon may reach almost grotesque proportions in some of the developing countries, where the introduction has been well described as follows:

'There are strong medical lobbies in these countries demanding urban hospitals, the most sophisticated equipment, foreign medical training and medical degrees from abroad, drugs with reputed Western name tags, and generally a preference for anything foreign, including medical journals and research. Not much attempt is being made to generate endogenous capacities in any sector of this broad spectrum. The medical elite is far too wedded to a Northern ethos of health' (Third World Forum Newsletters, March 1980, no. 5). This is completely true of psychiatry, whose principles and practice have been imported into developing countries from other societies.

Psychiatry has been 'patronised' by both the lay and professional classes of people in a way that is damaging to its reputation, partly because of its apparently 'non-scientific' methodology and partly because of the fact that it deals with a section of the community that is usually alienated from its culture.

It is important for the policy-makers and politicians to be re-educated to become aware of the fact that psychiatry has a preventive and mental health component and that its knowledge could contribute to better functioning of individuals and the community at large. Psychiatry, as an important area of medical care, could contribute to national and individual productivity. For example, schizophrenic disorders are essentially disorders of young people in their productive age and their cost to any action could be very high indeed. A cost/benefit analysis has shown clearly in some of the developing countries (cf. some of my findings in Aro, 1954–63) that a great deal of preventive and curative care could be provided at low cost by the total mobilisation of community resources, without sophisticated equipment or gigantic institutions, by using the services of nurses, social workers and many grades and cadres of auxiliaries, thereby making psychiatric care available widely to many people who are in need of it.

It is obvious that 'national will' and 'political will' must exist before a major improvement in the mental health services can be expected. Political decision-makers must have relevant information about the size and nature of mental health and broad psychosocial problems and methods for their solution as well as the social, economic and political gains to be expected from such improvement of mental health status of individuals and the community.

In a similar way, the politicisation of health in many of the developed countries has brought some advantages. With the investment in research, which until recently has been significant, the returns have been substantial and beneficial. The last three decades have seen a tremendous increase in research activities in biomedical sciences, aimed at finding answers to some of the great intellectual challenges that concern mankind as well as to the minimum needs of society. Molecular biologists and geneticists have brought about a biological revolution. Modern techniques of genetic engineering allow us to insert new genetic information into cells or transfer genetic material from one organism to another. These revolutionary advances hold out great promise, not only in the biological sciences, but also in general medicine, in agriculture and in industry.

Unfortunately, psychiatry, because of its historical evolution and its nature, has until now been isolated from this mainstream of fundamental and clinical research. This may be due partly to the fact that it has relied so much on psychological therapeutic methods such as psychoanalysis. It is therefore in a great measure the fault of psychiatrists themselves if they now find their discipline overtaken by the events in the mainstream of medical science. Very little investment has been made into psychiatric research, even though psychiatric disability increases and cripples the economy of nations and social life of individuals. Unfortunately, these facts remain hidden from the policy-makers and the politicians.

3. How do you regard the current emphasis on primary care in relation to psychiatric theory and practice?

There is no doubt that there is a wealth of knowledge accumulated by psychiatric theory and practice over the ages which could be applied to primary health care. The study of human development and social phenomena have given rise to a new psychobiological approach which has become a powerful tool designed purposely to bring together many disciplines – biological and social sciences – which could throw light on our understanding of man, his life reactions and his capacity for growth and development. In my opinion, a firm understanding of the life of the patient in his total environment, and the recognition of the role of the milieu in the development of the disease, should lead to a better insight into the total management of the patient. This dynamic conceptualisation formed the basis of Adolf Meyer's therapeutic principles and practice. Adolf Meyer subscribed to the dialectic position that the genuine objects of science are only the immediate observations and experiences themselves. This view supports the important role of psychiatry in primary health care.

The essential thrust of primary health care should be within the community, using all community resources for the prevention, treatment and rehabilitation of the psychiatrically ill. It is therefore necessary to enlarge the scope and obligation of psychiatry to encompass a multitude of social, biological, cultural and physical factors. It is for this reason that we need a mixed group of medical and health workers as well as practitioners of other disciplines, for example general practitioners, nurses, sociologists, teachers and educators, social workers, anthropologists, psychologists, behavioural scientists, possessing varying degrees of mental health skills and knowledge which could significantly improve the quality and effectiveness of mental health care and assistance. The application of our present-day knowledge derived from social and behavioural sciences could help us overcome some of the adverse effects of urbanisation, up-rooting and social disorganisation within the community, and also the other repercussions of socio-economic and technological changes which are taking place at a rapid rate in many societies today.

William James, in *The Energies of Man*, identified 'excitements, ideas, and efforts' as motivating forces for heightened energy. The evidence for these forces can be seen in such contemporary and dedicated groups as the Israeli Kibbutzim, Mao's Chinese social, cultural and political movements, and the Oneida Community, to mention only a few. Contemporary journals of psychology and other literature are full of accounts of the individual's triumphs over formidable external obstacles, emotional and physical handicaps, and situations of extreme stress, such as sensory deprivation and starvation. Here I refer to Bettelheim's clinical account of the overcoming of a concentration camp experience. The research of Miller and his colleagues (1971) on biofeedback and learned modifications of autonomic functions are equally relevant.

All these factors have implications for future educational principles concerning the growth and development programme of children in all cultures and societies. Any serious attempt to harness and transform human energy, create new ideals and bring about a new conception of human relations and a new understanding of individual and social responsibility will have to start with the education of children. The problem remains of how to generate exciting new developments in educational principles and to achieve an 'ideal' model of 'education' for the young in order to raise the human mind to a higher plane of activities.

It follows, then, that one of the objectives of education, as in therapy, is to generate and transcend wider and deeper here-and-now experiences, guided by a theory of man and of education which combines the charm of a child, the morality of a saint, the rigour of a scholar, the intuition of an artist and the maturity of a child-like adult. The approach, therefore, is to prompt responses of exploring areas that are not only immediately, but also latently, available for full development.

Nature, through the process of natural selection, has produced a man whose brain remains partially amorphous at birth. It is not the blank '*tabula rasa*' postulated by John Locke, nor are all its abilities innate, as Gobineau contended. Appropriate social, cultural and environmental experience is necessary at optimal periods for the stimulation of the embryonic genetic mechanisms to complete their tasks.

We must explore all possibilities that may exist to institute early warning and monitoring systems. We should also develop social indicators sensitive and sophisticated enough to identify individuals and families in distress; to ameliorate adverse social and material conditions and enhance the quality of life for those at the bottom of the social and economic pyramid; and to identify special high risk groups, such as children, migrants, refugees, minorities and people in transition. Value systems will continue to undergo enormous change and family roles will, of necessity, be modified. If man and his family are to remain syntonic with the emerging necessities in the changing milieu, the adequate design of interdisciplinary tools will have to be made to assist in this task and the emphasis will have to be at the primary care level.

References

Bolis, C. L. (1978*a*). WHO Neurosciences Programme for control of neurological disorders. *Trends in Neurosciences*, 1, no. 4, i–ii.

Bolis, C. L. (1978*b*). The WHO approach to neurological disorders. *Trends in NeuroSciences*, 1, no. 4, viii.

British Medical Journal (1980). The flight from science. *Br. Med. J.*, 280, 1.

Heisenberg, W. (1952). *Philosophical Problems of Nuclear Physics*, p. 107. Faber & Faber.

Jablensky, A., Sartorius, N., Gulbinat, W. & Ernberg, G. (1981). Characteristics of depressive patients contacting psychiatric services in four cultures – A report from the WHO collaborative study on the assessment of depressive disorders. *Acta psychiat. Scand.*, 63, 367–83.

James, W. (1907). The energies of Men. *Science*, *25*, 321–32.

Lambo, T. A. (1956). Neuropsychiatric observations in the Western Region of Nigeria. *Br. Med. J.*, ii, 1388–94.

Lambo, T. A. (1962). The influence of cultural factors on epidemiological surveys in Africa. *W. Afr. Med. J.*, 10, 87–92.

Lambo, T. A. (1965). Psychiatry in the tropics. *Lancet*, ii, 1119–21.

Lambo, T. A. (1975). 'Psychiatry's new challenges.' Address to the Annual Meeting of the American Psychiatric Association (Adolf Meyer Lecture), Anaheim, California, 6 May 1975. Geneva: WHO (mimeograph).

Lewis, A. (1958). Between guesswork and certainty in psychiatry. *Lancet*, i, 171–5.

Miller, N., Di Cara, L. & Solomon, H. (1971). *Biofeedback and self-control.* Aldine-Atherton, Chicago.

Rothman, T. (1962). In *The Future of Psychiatry*, ed. P. Hoch & J. Zubin, proceedings of the 51st Annual Meeting of the American Psychopathological Association. Grune & Stratton, New York.

Rowntree, J. W. (1949). *Claim Your Inheritance*, p. 107. Baumisdale Press.

Ryle, G. (1949). *The Concept of Mind*, p. 16. Hutchinson.

Sartorius, N. (1975). Epidemiology of depression. *WHO Chronicle*, **29**, 423–7.

Sartorius, N. (1980*a*). Research on affective psychoses within the framework of the WHO Programme. In *Prevention and Treatment of Affective Disorders*, Academic Press Inc. (London), pp. 208–13. Proceedings of a Symposium, Aarhus University, Denmark, August 1978.

Sartorius, N. (1980*b*). The research component of the WHO mental health programme. *Psychological Medicine*, 10, 175–85.

Sartorius, N., Jablensky, A., Gulbinat, W. & Ernberg, G. (1980). Application of WHO scales for the assessment of depressive states in different cultures. In *Epidemiological Research as Basis for the Organization of Extramural Psychiatry. Acta psychiat. scand., Suppl.* **285**, 62, 204–11.

Sartorius, N. & Jablensky, A. (1981). Collaborative research leading to guidelines for the treatment of depressive patients in developing countries. In *Rehabilitation of patients with schizophrenia and with depressions*, ed. J. K. Wing, P. Kielholz & W. M. Zinn, pp. 70–81. Hans Huber, Berne.

Third World Forum Newsletters (1980). March, no. 5.

World Health Organization (1973). *Report of the International Pilot Study of Schizophrenia*, Vol. 1, WHO, Geneva.

World Health Organization (1978*a*). The WHO Medium Term Mental Health Programme, 1975–1982. Interim Report. WHO, Geneva.

World Health Organization (1978*b*). Report on the Second Meeting of Investigators of the WHO Project on the Effects of Psychotropic Drugs in Different Populations. WHO, Geneva (offset document).

World Health Organization (1979). *Schizophrenia: an International Follow-Up.* John Wiley and Sons, Ltd.

Yap, P. M. (1951). Mental diseases peculiar to certain cultures (A survey of comparative psychiatry). *J. Ment. Sci.*, 97, 313–27.

Select bibliography

See also publications by T. A. Lambo in References, p. 120.

Lambo, T. A. (1955). The role of cultural factors in paranoid psychoses among the Yoruba tribe. *J. Ment. Sci.*, 101, 239–66.

Lambo, T. A. (1958). Psychiatric syndromes associated with cerebrovascular disorders in the African. *J. Ment. Sci.*, 104, 133–43.

Lambo, T. A. (1959). Mental health in Nigeria: research and its technical problems. *Wld. Ment. Hlth.*, **11**, 131–8; (1961) **13**, 135–41.

Lambo, T. A. (1960). Further neuropsychiatric observations in Nigeria (with comments on the need for epidemiological study in Africa). *Br. Med. J.*, ii, 1696–704.

Lambo, T. A. (1961). Schizophrenia-like psychoses associated with amphetamine intoxication in African students. *Dokita* no. 2, 33–7.

Lambo, T. A. (1961). Conference report of First Pan-African Psychiatric Conference, Abeokuta, Nigeria, 12–18 November 1961. Ibadan; Government Printer.

Lambo, T. A. (1962*a*). Malignant anxiety: a syndrome associated with criminal conduct in Africans. *J. Ment. Sci.*, **108**, 256–64.

Lambo, T. A. (1962*b*). The utilisation of environmental factors in psychiatric treatment. In: Transcultural studies panel discussion at the Third World Congress of Psychiatry, 10 June 1961. *Acta Psychiatrica Scand.*, **38**, 157–82.

Lambo, T. A. (1963). *African Traditional Beliefs, Concepts of Health and Medical Practice*. Inaugural lecture, Philosophical Society of the University of Ibadan. Ibadan University Press.

Lambo, T. A., Leighton, A. H., Hughes, C. C., Leighton, D. C., Murphy, F. M. & Macklin, D. B. (1963). *Psychiatric Disorders among the Yoruba. A Report from the Cornell–Aro Mental Health Research Project in the Western Region of Nigeria*. New York: Cornell University Press.

Lambo, T. A. (1964). The village of Aro. *Lancet*, ii, 513–14.

Lambo, T. A. (1965). Socio-economic changes in Africa and their implications for mental health. In *Man and Africa*, ed. G. Wolstenholme & M. O'Connor. London: Churchill-Livingstone.

Lambo, T. A. (1967). Mental and behavioural disorders. In *Health of Mankind*, ed. G. Wolstenholme & M. O'Connor. London: Churchill-Livingstone.

Lambo, T. A. (1968). Schizophrenia: its features and prognosis in the African. Inaugural speech. In *Deuxième Colloque Africain de Psychiatrie, Dakar, 5–9 Mars 1968*. Paris: Audecam.

Lambo, T. A. (1969). The child and the mother–child relationship in major cultures in Africa. *UNICEF Assignment Children* **10**, 61–74.

Lambo, T. A. (1971). *Human needs in the wake of rapid change in Africa*. Paper presented at the Conference on Cultural Relations for the Future Studies. Ibadan: Ibadan University (mimeograph)

Lambo, T. A. (1973). *Psychiatric research: world perspectives*. Paper presented at the 20th Anniversary Celebration of Rockland Research Center, New York, February 1973. Geneva: WHO (mimeograph).

Lambo, T. A. (1973). *Higher education in developing countries with emphasis on the concept of the international university*. Paper presented at the Second International Symposium on Transcultural Adaptation, Port au Prince, Haiti. Geneva: WHO (mimeograph).

Lambo, T. A. (1973). A world view of mental health: recent developments and future trends. Paper presented at the 1973 Presidential Session, American Orthopsychiatric Association Annual Meeting. *Am. J. Orthopsychiat.*, **43**, 706–16.

Lambo, T.A. (1973). *The challenge of change for developing countries*. Milton S. Eisenhower Lecture. Johns Hopkins University, Baltimore, Maryland. Geneva: WHO (mimeograph).

Lambo, T. A. (1974). The history of psychiatry in Mid and West Africa. In *World History of Psychiatry*, ed. J.G. Howells. New York: Brunner/Mazel, pp. 579–99.

Lambo, T. A. (1976). 'The promotion of health: the world situation.' Address to the Centenary Conference of the Royal Society of Health, London, November 1976.

Lambo, T. A. (1978). *Le Médecine-man dans la Tradition Africaine*. Prospective et Santé, No.5.

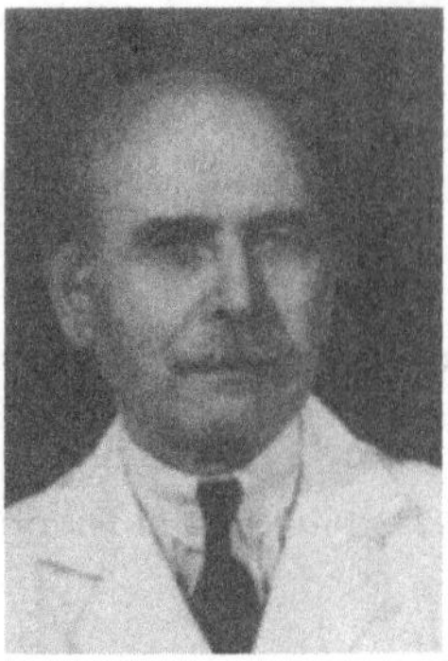

8 · PIERRE PICHOT

Personal background and professional experience

I was born on the 3 October 1918 at La Roche-sur-Yon in Vendée in the west of France. I received both my primary and my secondary classical education at Rennes in Brittany. My first inclination was to follow a scientific career, but the abstract nature of studies in the scientific schools of France caused me to turn instead to medicine. I have, however, always retained a predilection for historical studies and for languages that derives from my traditional classical education, as well as for mathematics, all of which have influenced my psychiatric preoccupations.

I went to Paris to study medicine because of the special prestige attached in France to the medical school there. I took the competitive examination for a training post in the Hospitals of Paris, which was and still is in France an essential requirement for anyone who has it in mind eventually to pursue a university career. In 1938 I was accepted as an externe and in 1944, after an interruption due to a period in the army, as an interne in the Hospitals of Paris. My interest lay then in neurology, which seemed to me at that time the pre-eminently scientific discipline, and I thought of returning to Brittany as a consultant. My teacher in neurology, Professor Alajouanine, advised me in these circumstances to acquire a complementary education in psychiatry and recommended me to Professor Jean Delay, who accepted me as an interne in his department. Shortly afterwards, Professor Delay suggested that I should abandon my original plans and stay on in Paris as his collaborator, with a view to taking up a university career in psychiatry. I can hardly claim, therefore, that psychiatry was my first vocational choice.

As soon as my mind was made up, I decided to widen my knowledge of the sciences that are ancillary to psychiatry. I studied general psychology at the Sorbonne under P. Guillaume, who introduced Gestalt psychology to France, and applied psychology at the Institute of Psychology in the University of Paris, where the orientation was towards methodology and statistics (factor analysis was taught there from 1945). These interests were reinforced by my secondment for some time to the army psychological service which, with the advice of the British army, was then engaged in preparing mental tests for use in the selection of soldiers and officers. I received my Doctorate of Medicine in 1948 and from then onwards I continued my psychiatric career at the Hospital of Sainte-Anne, where Jean Delay held the only Chair in Adult Psychiatry which existed in Paris at that time. I became Chief of Clinic in 1948 and then Assistant from 1949 to 1955, when I was made a Professor of Psychiatry. In 1964 I was given a Personal Chair in Medical Psychology and in January 1972 I succeeded Professor Delay as holder of the Chair in Clinical Psychiatry. Since 1948 I have also been responsible for a new course at the Institute of Psychology on statistical psychology applied to psychopathology, and for several years I have conducted a course in social applied psychology at the Sorbonne.

It is clear that the person who influenced me most in psychiatry was Jean Delay, to whom I acted successively as interne, Chief of Clinic, Assistant and Professor. Thanks to his high intelligence and the multiplicity of his interests, which ranged from neuropsychology to psychopathology and biological psychiatry, Jean Delay exerted a remarkable influence on the development of modern French psychiatry. The author of a classical treatise on astereognosia, and of the first comprehensive book on the EEG to appear in France, he also published notable works on the psychopathology of memory and of mood in the tradition of the French school exemplified by his teacher, Pierre Janet. Keenly interested also in psychobiology, he carried out numerous studies of electro-convulsive therapy and later of chemotherapy, the results of which are well known. He had himself undergone a training analysis, but although he succeeded in recruiting psychoanalysts into his department and made use of psychodynamic concepts in several of his publications, his general attitude towards psychoanalysis was always marked by a certain critical reserve.

One of the most striking features of Jean Delay's direction of the department at Sainte-Anne was the tolerance he displayed towards orientations in which he was not personally interested but which he considered important. He thus always encouraged me in my studies of experimental psychology applied to psychiatry and in my work on quantitative psychopathology, methodology and statistics. I consider that the atmosphere prevailing in his department was the dominant influence in my training. Associated with it, however, was another major influence, namely, that arising from my psychological studies, particularly at the Institute of Psychology, where my original leanings towards scientific disciplines were revived. As early as 1948 I had published work on mental tests in psychiatry, at a time when clinical psychiatrists in France scorned any appeal to quantification and statistics. Later – though by this time the climate had begun to change and (from the 1950s) the framework was that of psychopharmacology – I helped to introduce rating scales into France and to plead for scientific methodology in the conduct of clinical trials. As might have been expected, I was also interested in nosological problems at that time. I believe that this twofold influence, the school of Jean Delay and my training in methodology and statistics, sums up the origins of my orientation, although, of course, other and more peripheral factors have also affected some of my work and interests.

Current status of psychiatry

In the 35 years which have passed since my first contact with psychiatry, our discipline has changed considerably in several ways. I have always maintained contact with schools of psychiatry in other countries and these have been intensified since I assumed the functions of President of the World Psychiatric Association. The opinions which I am able to give on the present state of psychiatry, however, clearly relate in the first place to the situation in France. I shall deal successively with three areas which seem to me fundamental: the number of psychiatrists, the practice of psychiatry and the variety of orientations within the discipline.

The number of psychiatrists

The enormous increase in the number of psychiatrists since the last war is a striking phenomenon, especially in industrial countries such as France. There are many reasons for this rise: in the first place, there is the intellectual prestige that psychiatry has acquired outside medicine among the educated public, particularly because of the influence of psychoanalysis; there is also the social preoccupation of governments which consider that mental health should receive high priority in view of the number of patients and the cost involved, and which have therefore multiplied the number of public health posts in psychiatry and have given special privileges to medical students taking up the specialty (in France particularly since 1968). It must also be admitted, however, that in countries with liberal medical facilities this increase has applied even more to psychiatrists in private practice than to those in public health services, and it is moreover probable that the trend will soon cease, at least in countries in which there is now a high density of psychiatrists. It would seem that medical students are turning away from psychiatry: in the United States, for example, the proportion of those choosing this specialty dropped from 12 per cent in 1968 to less than 3 per cent in 1978. In addition, governments which bear, whether directly or not, the essential cost of expenditure on health estimate that such expenditure is now reaching a level in relation to the national income which it is difficult to exceed. For this reason, in France the government has taken the view that the number of psychiatrists in training is now excessive and has decided to reduce it summarily from 1983. This phenomenon of stagnation or regression in the demography of psychiatrists, which is likely to continue or to be accentuated, is a subject of current concern.

The practice of psychiatry

Theoretically, at least, there is little connection between the institutional practice of psychiatry in 1945 and the clinical practice of the present day. In the past clinical work in most countries was mainly conducted in special hospitals that were generally isolated and overcrowded and where the patients were usually detained against their will. This has been replaced by an 'open' psychiatry in which the patient's stay in hospital is usually voluntary and short, in which a large part of treatment is conducted in outpatient departments and in 'intermediary structures' (for example, day hospitals and hostels) and in which restoration of the patient to his natural milieu is held to be the ideal goal. Moreover, whereas previously authority was concentrated in the hands of the doctor, he is now only one element in a multidisciplinary therapeutic team in which psychologists and social workers occupy an equal position. There have been several contributory causes to this development, known variously as community psychiatry in the United States and 'district psychiatry' (psychiatrie de secteur) in France. They include a general 'anti-authoritarian' movement in the realm of ideas, which has found its ultimate expression to some extent in anti-psychiatry; humanitarian, social and political influences; facilities afforded by the effectiveness of pharmacotherapy (in reality the determining factor); the role of pressure groups of psychologists or sociologists seeking to remove psychiatry from medicine; and faith on the part of the health authorities in the economic benefits to be expected from the new arrangements.

This problem has often been approached emotionally and dogmatically, with no understanding in many countries of its pragmatic aspects. The success of such changes depends on three conditions: (i) an adequate infrastructure of personnel and institutions since, contrary to the claims put forward to governments by its protagonists, this type of psychiatry is more expensive than the traditional system; (ii) progress in psychopharmacology which, in spite of assertions to the contrary, is the *sine qua non* of successful functioning; and (iii) a tolerant attitude on the part of society towards deviants.

My own attitude to this question, which is crucial to the future of psychiatry, may be summed up in the following three propositions. (i) For a large proportion of psychiatric patients a policy of short spells of inpatient treatment in special departments situated in general hospitals, together with the creation of outpatient departments and 'intermediary structures', has been rendered both feasible and desirable by therapeutic progress. (ii) Liberalisation of the law in regard to the mentally ill and emphasis on their restoration to a natural milieu are desirable in principle; however, tolerance by society of deviants is probably much less than it is thought to be, and if pushed to the extreme these measures carry the risk of provoking violent reactions on the part of the public which will only lead to regression. The mentally ill are, of course, no different from other sick people from the medical point of view, but their disorders manifest themselves so often in social behaviour that it would be dangerous not to take this factor into account. (iii) The participation of psychologists and social workers is indispensable, but I am fundamentally opposed to removing psychiatry from medicine, a trend which I regard as the chief cause of the recent decline of interest in our specialty among medical students.

Psychiatric orientations

Psychiatry has always been marked by tensions between contradictory points of view. Should it adopt a medical model? Is it, to follow German terminology, one of the natural sciences? Are 'mental illnesses' diseases, or is there, on the contrary, a specific model which distinguishes psychiatry from the rest of medicine? Can mental anomalies be understood only by way of analysis of the interpersonal relationships between patient and doctor? Are behaviour and its deviations learned, the mind of man being at birth a *tabula rasa*, or are they innate, determined essentially by constitution and by genetic inheritance? Are the aetiological factors in psychiatry essentially psychological, social or biological? These large and fundamental questions are not independent of each other and give rise to many associated problems: the legitimacy of attempting to quantify mental phenomena, the dividing line between health and illness, the role of the psychiatrist in society, to mention but a few.

From the point of view of the movement of ideas, the period during which I was developing my psychiatric career is highly illuminating. I was able twice to participate in developments which were almost unparalleled. All in all, the intervention of political and ideological factors gave this era a colouring which was in some ways picturesque, in others deplorable, and at the same time – using the words with the necessary caution – fundamental discoveries were producing revolutionary changes.

By 1945 psychiatry in France had developed little in its general ideas over the previous 50 years. The model was medical and the only innovations that took place were a timid liberalisation and the introduction of biological methods of treatment, such as malaria therapy, insulin therapy and electro-convulsive therapy. Some young and 'politically progressive' psychiatrists did, it is true, emphasise the part played by social factors in aetiology and treatment. Psychoanalysis was also considered 'progressive' on an intellectual and non-political plane, but with only a small circle of adherents it was of no more than marginal importance. Today it is hard to imagine the shock of the encounter with psychiatry in the United States, which at that time was endowed with an extraordinary prestige. American psychiatry, which was then resolutely oriented towards psychoanalysis, was essentially dynamic, anti-nosological and psychologically inclined. Genetics had been discredited by National Socialism. In 1949 I accompanied an American colleague on a visit to the German psychiatric centres and met Kurt Schneider at Heidelberg. It was explained to us that the psychiatry of Kurt Schneider, like most representatives of German psychiatry in general since Kraepelin, expressed the reactionary pessimism which had led to fascism, and that the creation of an Institute of Psychoanalysis, with the assistance of funds from the Government of the United States, would help to make the German mentality more democratic. This anecdote takes on a certain piquancy today when Kurt Schneider, whose work has only recently been discovered in the United States, is now more widely quoted there than in Germany.

The wave of psychoanalysis broke over France from 1945 onwards, seducing first the young psychiatrists, then the psychologists, whose numbers multiplied from 1950, and the so-called educated public. It was accompanied by a radical anti-constitutionalism, by a dislike of nosography and by a widespread opposition to biology. Between 1950 and 1960 the 'cold war' exerted a curious influence on the situation. The ideas which emanated from the USSR were in some ways in agreement with those coming from the United States, although they were based on different principles, in particular on a denial of hereditary factors and on the infinite plasticity of the mind. However, in the USA psychoanalysis dominated the scene and mental disorders were attributed to individual elements in the family milieu. In the USSR, by contrast, psychoanalysis was regarded as a reactionary, idealist doctrine; Pavlovism was the obligatory pathogenic concept, and social aetiology was the only aetiology that was recognised in principle. It was even proclaimed that the psychoses, which were already said to be on the decrease, would disappear completely once a socialist society was definitively established.

Soviet ideas at that time influenced only the very small number of doctors in France who were politically committed. Most young psychiatrists took their ideas from America, though there was a very clear time lag. Up to the middle of the 1960s it was exceptional for professors of psychiatry to be analysts, and the university departments of psychiatry were, in general, medical, biological and nosological in their orientation. The events of 1968, both in the universities and in society in general, marked the zenith in France of the trend which had begun at the end of the war. The structure of the social services was modified; district psychiatry became the official doctrine; the teaching of psychiatry was separated radically from that of neurology, while at the same time pressure was exercised against the university centres; forces favouring sociology which could be called 'Marxist' (both anti-biological and anti-psychoanalytical) combined with forces favouring psychology (these were fundamentally psychoanalytical) in an attempt to remove psychiatry from medicine. The anti-psychiatric movement, whose influence in France turned out to be ephemeral, was a particular expression of this trend.

In fact, however, the apparent triumph of this doctrinal radicalism concealed the advance of an underlying but opposing trend which has been growing in strength for the last 15 years. The decisive turning point came in 1952 with the introduction of chemotherapy which, despite the resistance expressed towards it, forced psychiatrists to adopt a biological attitude. From 1960 onwards the United States, where the earlier trend had originated, showed signs of a reversal in orientation. Genetics regained its honoured place, nosology reappeared as the 'criterion of research' and became a matter of serious concern, behaviour therapy arose to compete with psychoanalysis, and at the same time ethology became fashionable and biological research made increasingly rapid advances. From the beginning of the 1970s the movement spread to France, though there was both a time lag and a considerable amount of inertia in the field of ideas. Psychoanalytical influence is thus still much stronger in France than in the United States. Nevertheless, the newer orientation is increasing in importance. It corresponds, moreover, to a general movement in scientific concepts, namely the dominant position now occupied by biology, especially molecular biology, and also in broader terms, at least in France, to an attitude which in other sectors finds expression in the views of what is called the 'New Right'. Despite much resistance, it seems clear to me that present attitudes tend more and more to be diametrically opposed to those which prevailed 25 years ago. It is, moreover, now fashionable to defend a psychiatry which is biological, relatively favourable to a constitutional approach and nosological. If psychotherapy is practised, its effectiveness must be demonstrated. Quantitative description of symptomatology is preferred to dynamic interpretation. *The American Diagnostic and Statistical Manual* (DSM III) is from this point of view an unmistakable sign. We are entering a new era.

Future prospects of psychiatry

Extrapolations are always dangerous. No one in 1948 could have predicted that within a few years we would see the appearance of neuroleptics and antidepressants. Discoveries whose nature and consequences we cannot imagine may, perhaps in the near future, bring modifications of equal importance. Up to the present the great innovations in our discipline have been the fruits of empiricism, sometimes based on false hypotheses: one may recall here the hypothesis of antagonism between schizophrenia and epilepsy and of the rise of electro-convulsive treatment which then showed itself to be an important method of treating depression. To take the field of biology, there is no doubt that the study of the biochemistry of the brain and of neuro-transmitters holds out much promise, but the research so far conducted has been more useful in pointing the way to further research than in producing fundamental discoveries. Finally, one must not forget the role which will possibly be played by the application to psychiatry of techniques and ideas developed in completely different contexts.

From another perspective, the evolution of psychiatry, the extension of research and the improvement of patient care in medicine generally – but more particularly in psychiatry than in the 'organic' specialities – are all bound by economic factors to the social system. We know that the proportion of the national revenue devoted to expenditure on health is a reflection of society's values. This sum of money, which was negligible or almost negligible in the eighteenth century, is now very considerable. The current position, curiously expressed in WHO's proclamation of the 'right to health', is inevitably a matter of balance with other values. It probably depends less than we think on technical possibilities. At present it would be possible for the entire budget of a nation, no matter how prosperous, to be spent on ensuring that its citizens receive the best care that is available in the present state of our knowledge. Clearly this never happens. Moreover, within medicine psychiatry is often regarded as a 'luxury' specialty in developing countries, which in fact means for the majority of the world's population. In addition to the fact that tolerance of deviant behaviour is generally greater than in developed countries, there are also needs which claim high priority, such as the fight against malnutrition due to lack of protein in the diet or against parasitic diseases. There is no doubt that psychiatry in these developing countries, at least such psychiatry as is not reserved in practice for a particular 'westernised' and economically favoured group, will accompany advances in economic development. In industrial countries, on the other hand, the evolution of psychiatry cannot be predicted with the same certainty, since it will depend largely on changes in the value systems of nations and of governments, which are related to political attitudes in the broad sense.

Although it is easy to agree that psychiatry is one discipline, it contains three distinct components which, while not absolutely separate one from another, differ in their conditions of practice and their choice of treatment, and possible also in their prevailing concepts of aetiology and pathogenesis. Carrying this categorisation to its extreme one might say that there is first, a 'minor' psychiatry for neuroses, personality disorders and, speaking more generally, for the fringes of normality. Treatment is typically conducted outside the hospital milieu, and in certain countries is principally a matter of private practice; aetiology and pathogenesis are generally considered to be psychological and the main treatment is some form of psychotherapy or perhaps, in general practice for example, mild chemotherapy. Secondly, there is a psychiatry for the functional psychoses: practice here is mixed, taking place both within and outside the hospital milieu and resembling more the practice of 'organic' medicine; treatment is mainly by chemotherapy, while psychotherapy and sociotherapy are, in fact if not in theory, ancillary measures. Aetiology and pathogenesis are increasingly viewed as biological and it is here that most current psychiatric research is being carried out. Thirdly, there is a psychiatry for chronic defect states, oligophrenias, schizophrenic deficits and dementias. Treatment is conducted almost entirely within the hospital milieu and is little more than institutional in nature, with a small complement of chemotherapy; aetiology and pathogenesis are recognised as being organic.

Effort and attention in research have been concentrated preferentially on one or other of these forms of psychiatry, according to the period in question. The institutional asylum of the nineteenth century was centred on the third component, since the first was recognised only in its extreme forms and there was no treatment for the functional psychoses. During the 1950s the psychiatric model in the United States concentrated on the first component, the second being partially assimilated, explained and treated on the same lines (psychodynamic concepts and psychotherapy of the psychoses), and partly grouped with the third component. Psychiatry today is clearly concentrated on the second sector, that of the functional psychoses, both from the therapeutic point of view (inpatient departments in general hospitals for short-stay patients, with the possibility, thanks to chemotherapy, of at least temporary social rehabilitation) and from the point of view of the kind of research now in vogue concerning the biological basis of the psychoses. 'Minor' psychiatry tends to be conducted more and more by psychologists or entrusted to general practitioners. As for the psychiatry of those suffering from defect states, the tendency is for government projects to forget their existence, in spite of the problems they pose. The evolution of psychiatry must in any optimistic view of future perspectives try to achieve a balance between the three components, with no systematic favouring of one at the expense of the others.

The attitude adopted towards psychiatry can be seen both in the amount of economic investment in clinical and research work and in the administrative and legal measures taken to deal with the mentally ill. This attitude on the part of governments is largely a reflection of the attitude of the general public whom they represent. While not accepting the conclusions of Michel Foucault, according to whom the institutional psychiatry of the nineteenth century (the asylum system) was the expression of a bourgeois system of values, I would agree with him that there is a correspondence between attitudes to psychiatry and the general public's system of values (and in consequence political opinion in the broad sense). Quite apart from the drastic example of this interdependence which was provided by National Socialism, it seems clear that political 'liberalism' is correlated, temporally and geographically, with a loosening of the social restraints imposed upon patients (for example, confinement in hospital), with the 'psychiatrisation' of delinquent and more generally deviant forms of behaviour, and with a favourable attitude towards psychosocial therapies. Objective conditions doubtless also play a part: the change from the extended to the nuclear family as the dominant structure makes admission to hospital indispensable for senile dements, and the increasing complexity of work in an industrial society has progressively modified the limits between normality and mental deficiency. But without minimising the effect of these influences, it must be said that many decisions depend on choices which, in fact, have no connection with rational arguments. The introduction of community psychiatry in the United States or of district psychiatry in France was not preceded by any demonstration of their economic and/or therapeutic superiority. It would be a mistake to believe that this trend is irreversible because in the last 100 years the field of psychiatry has been extended to cover areas that formerly belonged to law, to religion or to ethics, and because there has been a liberalisation of the social measures adopted in relation to the mentally ill. Positions such as those taken up by men like Szasz, in spite of their extreme nature, bear definite witness to the existence of trends in the opposite direction.

Questions and answers

1. It is widely believed that psychiatry in France has tended to evolve in its own way, as exemplified by Professor Manfred Bleuler's recent comment, that 'French psychiatrists conceived a particular psychiatric classification in which a place for the concept of schizophrenia is difficult to find.' How do you regard this trend in the light of the increasing importance attached by the scientific community to international collaboration?

It is very widely held that the French system of nosology is idiosyncratic and does not conform to international concepts. In fact, all national schools whose tradition goes back a long time tend to be just as conservative, even if, unlike France, the originality of their underlying concepts is masked by the use of a common vocabulary. The area of schizophrenia, cited by Manfred Bleuler, is, moreover, the only one in which French psychiatry retains its own terminology (for example, *délires chroniques*, chronic delusions; *bouffées délirantes*, delusional outbursts). The explanation must be sought in terms of historical evolution. The French school occupied a dominant position during the first two-thirds of the nineteenth century and was, from the 1850s, inspired by Morel's doctrine of mental degeneration. Towards 1900 the accepted nosology was that of Magnan, who had carried the concept of degeneration a stage further. Kraepelin's ideas then came on the scene, and there are some historians who see in the war of 1870 a symbolic landmark signalling France's cession to Germany of the dominant position in psychiatry. Without going into details of a history which has been traced by Bonfils ('Histoire du concept de démence précoce en France', Thèse de médecine, Paris 1979), I would agree with him that 'it is because [French psychiatrists] were wedded to the concept of degeneration that the notion of dementia praecox as we know it today could not take root in France and it is for the same reason that the Kraepelinian concept of dementia praecox dealt a mortal blow to classical French psychiatry'. In practice, a compromise was finally reached in which Kraepelin's categories were partly accepted, followed by Bleuler's (the hebephrenic, catatonic and paranoid forms of schizophrenia) but as much as possible of the classical categories was retained: the 'chronic delusions' with their special forms were removed from paranoid schizophrenia, and the 'delirious outbursts of degenerates' were removed from the acute states which Bleuler had once more grouped with schizophrenia. The use of an original and traditional vocabulary (chronic hallucinatory psychosis, delusion of interpretation, delusion of passion, delusion of imagination or paraphrenia for the 'chronic delusions' and for the acute states) has lent an exotic colouring to this nosology. But in fact 'delusional outbursts' are described by DSM III as schizophreniform psychoses, which likewise lie outside the category of schizophrenia.

2. As President of the World Psychiatric Association, what do you think this body can do to further the development of psychiatry?

The World Psychiatric Association (WPA) was born of a decision taken at the end of the last war by a group of French psychiatrists headed by Jean Delay and Henri Ey to organise an International Congress of Psychiatry in

Paris in 1950. The aim was to show that psychiatry had become a major medical discipline, independent of neurology and, further, not to be confused with preoccupations with 'mental health' which to a large extent carries a wider connotation than medicine. From this arose the WPA, which has progressively come to include almost all the existing psychiatric societies in the world today. The means by which the WPA pursues its aims are the organisation of world congresses every five or six years, of regional symposia, which are limited geographically but take place more frequently, and of technical symposia run by special sections. The existence of other international groups concerned with particular areas in psychiatry, or particular theoretical orientations (biological, psychological or social), or particular technical fields, creates an impression of competition with the WPA. But the WPA has a specific mission which was formulated at the first Congress: to make psychiatrists, whatever their nationality, their special interests, their orientation or their technical level, aware of the specific nature of their discipline and of the common scientific bases on which it rests. By its nature it is the only body which can fulfil these aims. The justification for its present and future existence is that it is the guardian of psychiatric unity.

This ecumenical vocation implies that internal conflicts must be resolved. There are centrifugal factors in the WPA which are common enough in any medical association but which should not exert a long-term influence: ambitions on the part of groups struggling to establish one particular doctrine at the expense of others, contamination of legitimate scientific arguments by attempts to assert national power. The only serious confrontations which the WPA has known during the last few years, however, have been concerned with ethical problems. The practice of psychiatry is governed by the moral laws common to all medicine, but specific problems arise in psychiatry because its subject matter comprises disorders of behaviour and because its methods of treatment have, in consequence, an effect on behaviour. Two themes which are closely interwoven are thus brought to the fore: the dividing line between normal and pathological behaviour and the legitimacy of giving a doctor a part to play in social control, an issue of particular concern to psychiatrist as the the only doctor who is authorised to impose restrictions on the liberty of his patients.

3. Regarding the future of psychiatry in industrialised countries you say 'it will depend largely on changes in the value systems of nations and of

governments, which relate to political attitudes in the broad sense'. Could you indicate more precisely what you have in mind?

Some criticisms of psychiatric ethics and some demands for their modification are of a general nature. To quote two current examples, it may be urged that the psychiatrist should play no part in depriving a patient of his liberty, or that he should not have the right to treat a patient without his consent. Other criticisms have long been concerned with individual deviations, it being said that the psychiatrist does not respect the ethical rules accepted by all his medical colleagues: the classical case is that of 'arbitrary commitment'. But the most delicate problem, since it reflects internal disputes in psychiatry, refers to allegations according to which certain psychiatrists, because they belong to a particular social or national group, violate ethical rules that are universally accepted. Such allegations sometimes take the form of vague accusations: it is claimed that the psychiatrist judges social adaptation according to the interests of the class to which he belongs or which he serves. At other times the criticism is more circumscribed: for about 50 years there has been talk of psychiatrists participating in the development of methods of interrogation, within the framework of civil or international wars. Allegations of this kind have multiplied during recent years, and have been concerned chiefly with the internment in psychiatric hospitals of people whose behaviour is deviant according to the norms of the country in question but whose deviance is not of a pathological nature. This problem, known as 'the abuse of psychiatry for political ends', has received wide publicity. The WPA has served as a privileged arena for these debates, the seriousness of which is increased by the fact that the psychiatrists making the allegations and those who are accused of participating in such violations of accepted ethics belong to countries which differ fundamentally in their social and political ideologies. I have no illusions about the gravity of this situation so far as the future of the WPA is concerned. As I have already stated, the essential mission of the WPA is to maintain the unity of psychiatry and this unity relates equally to scientific doctrine and to national appurtenances. The member societies of our Association must realise that the loss of universality would deprive the WPA of the very reason for its existence. The future of the WPA depends on the manner in which its members are able to show, in their examination of ethical problems, the objectivity and wisdom which are the qualities that ought to be the hallmark of every psychiatrist.

Select bibliography

Pichot, P. (1948). *Les Tests Mentaux et Psychiatrie*. Paris: Presses Universitaires de France.

Pichot, P. (1954). *Les Tests Mentaux*. Paris: Presses Universitaires de France. (Translated into Czech, Iranian, Portuguese and Spanish.)

Pichot, P. (1955). *Méthodes Psychométriques en Clinique*. Paris: Masson et Cie.

Pichot, P., Delay, J., Lempérière, T. & Perse, J. (1955). *Le Test de Rorschach et la Personnalité Épileptique*. Paris: Presses Universitaires de France. (Translated into English.)

Pichot, P. & Delay, J. (1962). *Abrégé de Psychologie*. Paris: Masson et Cie. (Translated into German, Italian, Portuguese and Spanish.)

Pichot, P., Guelfi, J. & Hakim, C. (1972–3). *La Personnalité*. Paris: Roger Dacosta. (Translated into Spanish.)

Pichot, P. (1978). *Les Voies Nouvelles de la Dépression*. Paris: Masson et Cie.

Pichot, P. (1981). *Actualités de la Schizophrenie*. Paris: Presses Universitaires de France.

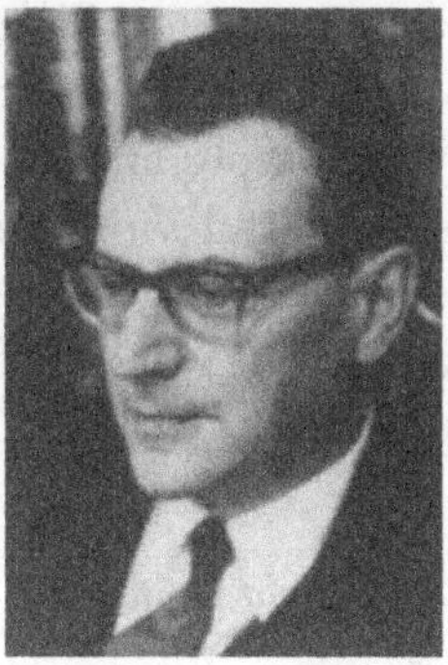

9 · JOHN ROMANO

Personal background and professional experience

Early Interests

As a medical student I was seriously interested in a number of career possibilities, including internal medicine, neurology and orthopaedic surgery, but in spite of the fact that the poorest teaching was done in the field of psychiatry, or perhaps because of it, I began to point my career towards this end. There were no courses in psychology or psychiatry in the pre-clinical period. As third-year medical students we had had two brief visits to the county mental hospital, during one of which I had the sobering experience of being assigned to a patient who had been a classmate of mine in high school many years before. He had been ill continuously for a period of seven years and was considered a chronic schizophrenic. I had a sickening sense of human inertia and illness in seeing so many patients just sitting and staring into space, but what disturbed me most was the presence of my former classmate. Someone whom I knew had become mad and remained socially disabled all those years. It was my introduction to chronic illness as well as to mental illness.

With another classmate, at the end of the third year in medical school, I was assigned to serve as a student extern at the Milwaukee County Asylum for Chronic Mental Diseases (1932–3). The patient population (about 1,500) was exclusively that of chronically ill persons, for the most part suffering from dementia praecox, but there were also epileptic patients with psychoses, other patients with irreversible rut depressions, those with persistent manic excitement and a considerable number with organic brain diseases, senile dementia and residual general paresis. We saw no harshness or cruelty, but were deeply impressed with the ambience of monotony, apathy and anonymity and with the fact that so many patients seemed to have been abandoned. During this period my classmate and I read from several current American textbooks of psychiatry, and also read Brill's translation of Eugen Bleuler's text of 1924 (Romano, 1977*a*).

Psychiatric Education

My first formal experience in the field was as an intern and resident in clinical psychiatry at Yale (1934–5). Eugen Kahn, Sterling Professor of Psychiatry and Mental Hygiene, had been at Yale for four years when I went there in 1934. Educated at Heidelberg, Berlin and Munich, where he received his Doctor of Medicine in 1911, Kahn spent the following 18 years on the staff of the University Psychiatric Clinic in close association with Professor Emil Kraepelin. I learned from Kahn not only of Kraepelin but also of the contributions of other continental psychiatrists. Particular emphasis was placed on Kretschmer's body type notions. I learned, too, of the attempts of Rudin to study schizophrenia according to Mendelian principles.

While Kahn represented traditional continental clinical psychiatry, the clinical conferences and patient presentations touched on many conceptual points of view and therapeutic approaches. I enjoyed meeting and knowing a number of persons who participated in our clinical conferences. Raymond Dodge, then Professor of Psychology in the Institute of Human Relations, told us of his earlier work with Diefendorf on the visual fixation of schizophrenic patients. Marian Cabot Putnam had just come to New Haven from her work with Anna Freud in Vienna, and Erik Homburger Erickson came several times after visiting the Dionne quintuplets. Roy Grinker visited us on his return from Vienna en route to Chicago, and talked to us about his psychoanalysis with Sigmund Freud. I learned much from Lloyd J. Thompson, who was well-versed in both diagnosis and treatment, and from Edwin J. Gildea, who conducted liaison teaching rounds on the surgical services and ran the biochemistry laboratory in the Department of Psychiatry. One of his major interests was studying the relations between blood lipids and constitutional body types. His laboratory provided an opportunity for me to set up assays of bromides and barbiturates in blood and urine.

It was years later that I realised that I had been deprived of the opportunity to know a number of distinguished scholars who were literally within bare-headed distance of the psychiatric hospital floor. Regrettably, the organisation, or perhaps the lack of such, of the Institute of Human Relations at Yale had led to the separation of the Psychiatric Department from Psychology and the Social Sciences, and so I did not get to know Ernest Sapir, John Dollard, Rollo May, Neal Miller and others.

I read as extensively and as wisely as I knew, but I learned more from my day-to-day experiences with my patients and their families and from the intimate exchange of ideas and experiences with the senior members of the house staff. I had become familiar with the several etiological models – genetic, biological and psychosocial – and tried to learn how each could help me in understanding my patient's behaviour. Because of the influence of Kahn, the Yale experience resembled more the setting of the continental university department of psychiatry than it did the American clinic at that time.

In the three years which followed (1935–8) I served as a Commonwealth Fund Fellow in Psychiatry in the University of Colorado where Franklin Ebaugh had brought the teachings of Adolf Meyer. Edward Billings, with the generous help of the Rockefeller Foundation, had just launched the medical–psychiatric liaison programme in the Colorado General Hospital, the University teaching hospital in Denver. John Benjamin had recently arrived from Zurich and from his association with the Bleulers and with Emil Oberholzer; he shared with us his interest and knowledge of psychoanalysis and the Rorschach test. He also gave us some idea of the general temper of continental psychiatry and was particularly interested in the cognitive disturbances of schizophrenic patients. It was principally through Henry Brosin that I learned more about the contributions of Adolf Meyer.

While the major thrust of the programme was our daily engagement in the study, care and treatment of patients and meetings with their families, we were also exposed to and involved in consultative services to courts and social agencies; in conducting demonstration child and adult clinics in several small towns in Colorado; in diagnostic and treatment services to a nearby institute for delinquent boys; in four- to five-month assignments to the large state hospital in Pueblo; in numerous public educational lectures to parent/teacher and lay organisations concerned with mental health in Denver and throughout the state. There was little or no formal instruction as we know it today in the form of tutorials, seminars, conferences or lectures. We taught and learned from each other, and at times our debates about the study, understanding and most appropriate care for our patients were long and heated. We vied with each other for assignments in the teaching of medical students (Romano, 1970).

There was little formal investigative work. One must remember that there were few scientific investigators who could serve as models. Psychiatry had no Rockefeller Institute to groom its young professors, as was the case in medicine and physiology. We had to wait almost 15 years before the National Institute of Mental Health became a reality. However, a number of us did become involved in clinical case studies, including prognostic studies in schizophrenia. I used the association motor test derived from the work of Alexander Romanovich Luria, whom I met later in Moscow. With Reuben Gustavson, then Professor of Chemistry at Denver University, we conducted studies of the excretion of oestrogenic and gonadotropic hormones in the urines of non-pregnant women, both in health and during manic excitements.

We were involved in the enthusiasms of the time, with continuous narcosis, insulin, the use of the Kettering Hypertherm in the treatment of patients with neurosyphilis, as well as with the more traditional psychotherapeutic techniques of the day. The sulphonamides had just arrived, but penicillin was yet to come, and we were to wait another 20 years before chlorpromazine was available. Later in our work metrazol was employed and ECT was on the horizon. Psychology and social work were represented by only a few valiant workers who served principally as handmaiden technicians. It was a far cry from the rich and profitable interchange that exists today with psychology and social work in most of the university departments.

Here again, the intellectual ambience of the department was eclectic, that is, pluralistic in the sense of considering the genetic, biological, psychological and social determinants of behaviour. In contrast to New Haven, we learned much more about the administrative organisation of mental health services in the community and in the state as a whole and, because of the liaison programme in our sister general teaching hospital, productive and harmonious relations were established with the other clinical departments.

For some time I had planned to obtain further systematic training in neurology and was pleased to be given a Rockefeller Fellowship at the National Hospital, Queen Square, London. Because of the imminence of the European war (September 1938), I chose to transfer the fellowship to the Harvard Neurological Unit at the Boston City Hospital (1938–9). It was an interesting time, as Tracy Putnam and Houston Merritt had just introduced the use of dilantin in the treatment of epileptic patients, and innovative surgical methods were being used to relieve the distress of patients with dystonia. I chose not to work on a special problem in order to spend my entire time seeing patients in neurological consultations. Together with the Chief Resident in Neurology (who had had psychiatric training), we would see some 10 to 12 new patients daily, referred to us from all the other clinical services in a large city general hospital. Three-quarters of the patients whom we were asked to see were those with predominantly psychiatric problems, presenting the differential diagnosis of many types of organic brain disease and delirium due to infection, trauma, alcohol, tumours, and other forms of cerebral pathology. Some patients exhibited attacks of acute anxiety; more demonstrated old-fashioned monosymptomatic hysterical behaviour. As I look back on it, the fellowship in neurology was an invaluable experience. In addition to broadening my knowledge of clinical medicine, neurology and psychiatry, it furthered my interest in the study of the delirious patient and also provided a psychosocial moratorium, a much-needed period for reflection and for an overview of the field.

Because I spent a great deal of time on the clinical floors in medicine and surgery, I met Soma Weiss, Harvard Professor of Medicine, then engaged in clinical research in the famous Thorndike Memorial Research Laboratory, an enclave in the Boston City Hospital. Weiss had just been appointed the Hersey Professor of the Theory and Practice of Physic and Chief of Medicine at the Peter Bent Brigham Hospital, the oldest chair of medicine at Harvard. Weiss picked Eugene Stead, Charles Janeway and myself to constitute his new full-time faculty in medicine at the Peter Bent Brigham Hospital (1 September 1939). My assignments were to be responsible for the development of teaching programmes and research in the fields of neurology and psychiatry.

It was a dramatic moment in time. Hitler had bombed Warsaw the very day that Stead, Janeway and I joined Soma Weiss to start the new department of medicine (September 1939). The hospital had no formal inpatient psychiatric service but, when necessary, I hospitalised psychiatric patients for short periods on the medical or surgical floors. I conducted psychiatric and neurological outpatient clinics, and much of my assignment was in consultative work on the medical and surgical floors of the hospital. It was here that I began a more systematic study of delirious patients and also began a study of patients with several types of psychosomatic illnesses, including duodenal ulcer, thyroid disease and ulcerative colitis. I learned much about preparation for surgery and the emotional problems of surgical patients (Romano, 1979). This experience gave me full opportunity to know something of the psychiatric problems in a university teaching general hospital, and particularly about death and dying.

I was interested in obtaining more experience in the field of psychoanalysis and, together with George Gardner and Charles Brenner, I was appointed Sigmund Freud Fellow in Psychoanalysis in the Boston Psychoanalytic Institute (September 1939). In addition to the personal analysis, I began attending the various seminars conducted by Isador Coriat, Helene and Felix Deutsch, Greta and Edward Bibring, Jenny and Robert Waelder, M. Ralph Kaufman, Ives Hendrick, Marian Cabot Putnam (who had come to Boston from New Haven) and others.

My early expectations of the influence of psychoanalytic psychology on clinical psychiatry have been modified by further experience. In 1950 I stated, '... psychiatry, particularly through psychoanalytic psychology, will play a major role in the scientific humanization of biology ... '. In 1961 I was to modify this view: 'Though the contributions of psychoanalytic psychology have been of inestimable value in providing a conceptual scheme of mind or mental apparatus, it obviously cannot serve as a general psychology, much less as a satisfactory approach to a human biology inclusive of social concepts.' Later still I reflected: 'Perhaps our experience over the past 25 years with several psychoanalytic institutes in other communities will not be repeated in the future – I sincerely hope it will not. With the exception of the Chicago Institute, which, under the leadership of Franz Alexander and Thomas French, did exhibit interest in scholarship for itself, most others with whom we dealt in working with associations for educational purposes reflected the narrowness and the arrogance of those who maintain closed systems of belief and practice' (Romano, 1975). However, there is little question that dynamic psychotherapy, as influenced by psychoanalytic psychology, has had a tremendous humanising influence on all of medicine. It has helped inestimably in the understanding of one another and our patients, and has made possible the beginning of a systematic approach to studying the interaction between patient and physician. Our increasing concern with the human family as well as the human community has added immeasurably to our understanding of the human condition.

In the two University Departments where I have served as Chairman we have maintained the belief that the major function of the psychiatrist, and one unique to him, is that he serves as a crucial bridge between genetics, biology and clinical medicine on one hand, and the behavioural sciences on the other. In my Salmon Lecture, delivered in 1976, I said:

The psychologist, the social worker, and the social scientist lack knowledge of the body, the biologist that of the mind, and up to the present, the nurse has had insufficient scholarship in either field to serve the purpose of a bridge. Further, I believe that if we are to serve this function properly, we must become expert in both biologic and psychosocial systems. Only then will we be able to interrelate effectively the knowledge from these basic sources in our unique role and contribution as clinician and scientist. To neglect scholarship at either pole would be to diminish our usefulness for tomorrow. While we may derive knowledge from the biology and psychosocial systems, we must also contribute to them. We can do this best in our historic and essential role as psychiatric clinicians.

Current status of psychiatry

It is generally agreed that the profession has achieved a number of goals set by it more than 35 years ago. It is also agreed that there remain goals yet to be achieved.

We have fulfilled our expectations in effecting an increase of professionals (from 2 psychiatrists per 100,000 population in 1935 to over 12 per 100,000 in 1979); in the education of our medical students; in introducing psychology and the social sciences into the matrix of the medical school; in the establishment of psychiatric units in general hospitals; in the pursuit of research in biological and physicochemical, as well as psychological and social, fields; in the treatment of the acutely ill psychotic patient; in increasing public awareness of the prevalence of mental distress and the provision of community services for study and care. Whatever we have accomplished we do need to do better, and there is much left to be done.

We have yet to achieve an effective relationship with the law and the courts. We need clarification and enhancement of our professional roles with our colleagues in the departments of the medical school and in the university at large. Regrettably, there has been continued neglect of the chronic psychiatric patient and, what is more serious, limited understanding of the burden of dependency carried by the families of our patients.

Nonetheless, in spite of the goals achieved, in whole or in part, one hears or reads that psychiatry is dead, or at least dying, and that its great days are past. Much of what may be past or passing is the more limited professional role which psychiatrists played earlier in the century. We are more numerous, more diverse in function, and society calls upon us to respond to many needs, for some of which we are not equipped. The parallel exponential increase in non-medical professionals and para-professionals now engaged in mental health services has led to a fragmentation of the traditional functions of the psychiatrist. Predictably, this has resulted in some confusion on the part of the psychiatrist as to his professional role. One often hears or reads of psychiatrists who ask, 'Who am I? What knowledge and which skills shall I need in my professional work? Who will be my patients, and with whom do I share responsibility for the sick?'

Role confusion is further intensified by the explosive multiplication of psychotherapeutic modes (in great part generated by non-psychiatrists), but due mainly to disappointments with the effectiveness of traditional psychotherapy. In turn, this has led to indiscriminate, and at times irresponsible, treatment of the sick and the non-sick, practices often attributed to the psychiatrist.

An unfortunate sequel to the community mental health movement in America has been the uncritical, naive and passive obeisance of the psychiatric profession in embarking on ambitious and, at times, grandiose clinical service programmes without insisting on systematic and appropriate trial, and without adequate financial support from state or local funds. Along with this trend there has been an increasing intrusion into the daily practice of the psychiatrist by governmental and judicial agencies, with a consequent erosion of his traditional clinical authority and subsequent responsibility in the care of the sick entrusted to him.

While remarkable changes have certainly taken place in the profession since the introduction of anxiolytic, neuroleptic and anti-depressant medication, the unfortunate and shameful fact remains that many psychiatrists, poorly versed in psycho-pharmacology, prescribe these drugs unwisely and at times haphazardly.

There is much to applaud in our renewed interest in the care and treatment of psychotic patients and in the changes which have brought about greater intimacy between the chronic hospitals and the communities which they serve. We should be pleased, too, with our increased interest in genetics and in studies of the biochemical and physiological aspects of brain and mind, but there is little to be proud of in our continuing neglect of chronically ill patients both in the hospital and in the community.

Whether our concerns differ in kind or number from those of our predecessors in other times and places will be decided by tomorrow's historians. Several colleagues have commented that this confusion as to our identity, which many believe to be the pervasive problem of the day, has been recognised as a problem among psychiatrists since at least World

War II, if not before. They point out that similar confusion exists in the psychiatric professions of other nations. It is said that each generation is apt to overestimate its contribution to its society and, perhaps for the same reasons, to overestimate the seriousness of its problems.

Future prospects of psychiatry

Although there are still many problems to be solved, I see no need to chant a requiem mass for the repose of the soul of psychiatry. Rather, it is time to sound a reveille to call the profession to rise and fulfil our professional responsibility more effectively.

I continue to believe that a major area of unfinished business is a search for that which is basic and essential to the psychotherapeutic encounter. Psychiatrists – with their colleagues in psychology, biology and the social sciences – must pursue with increasing vigour those studies which one day may enable us to act less blindly and to prescribe the appropriate therapy to help our patients. There is so much more for the psychiatrist to learn about this very influential phenomenon which takes place between the patient (the one who suffers) and the physician (the one who wishes to help). This has been the thread of continuity, the means of survival, of the physician throughout the centuries, regardless of how informed or uninformed and how helpful or harmful he has been to those who sought his aid.

We must clarify our roles and the roles of others, both professional and para-professional, who share in the study, care and treatment of the sick and their families. Our present deceptive egalitarianism has led to confusion worse confounded and, in practice, has led to the lowest common denominator of skill. We should cease to act blindly as self-appointed social engineers–saviours, and learn from experiment and trial whether and how our skills and knowledge are applicable to social issues.

More recently, in reviewing our position over the past 45 years in the teaching of psychiatry to medical students, I listed a number of factors which may be responsible for the current decline in the number of medical students who choose psychiatric careers. In my view, the major factor among several others is the downgrading of the teaching of psychiatry to medical students. As I go about the country, I find very few senior faculty members working intimately with the medical students. I wondered whether we fouled our own nest by permitting, even fostering, a teaching programme which can no longer compete with the excitement and promise of our sister clinical disciplines. Have we uncritically embraced an anti-authoritarianism which has diminished quality in all of our undertakings and which has led to the breakdown of our previous standards?

In concluding this commentary on the teaching of medical students, I tried to summarise my position as follows:

> If we can recreate the ambiance of the imaginative acquisition of knowledge, if our students see about them residents, interns, faculty (junior and senior) who exhibit and enjoy the great excitement and richness of our field, the most human, the most personal of the medical disciplines; if there are those who retain their curiosity, wish to know more and wish to apply their knowledge for the benefit of those who seek their help, and if they consider their primary allegiance to be to the problem that the patient and the patient's family present rather than to their own private ideologies, we may not only assure our survival but actually continue to grow. This will mean comprehensive understanding of genetic and biologic as well as psychosocial determinants, the intelligent use of medication when indicated; identifying the type of psychotherapy appropriate to the patient's needs and the use of community resources beyond the family when indicated. If we can achieve these objectives, we may again earn the respect of others, most particularly the respect of our students. If not, there may be no good reason for us to survive as a major medical discipline (Romano, 1980).

Questions and answers

1. In view of the post-war upsurge of interest in psychiatry in American medical schools how do you account for the current 'downgrading of the teaching of psychiatry to medical students' to which you refer?

Regrettably, there is neglect of the teaching of medical students throughout the clinical curriculum. The matter is complex, but because of compelling financial stringencies many, if not most, full-time clinical teachers must now 'sing for their supper'. This means that they must see sufficient numbers of private patients in order to ensure their salaries. As a consequence, teaching, even more than research activities, is sacrificed, particularly the teaching of medical students. This downgrading of teaching is clearly evident in psychiatry. Few senior full-time professorial psychiatrists work intimately with medical students. The financial reason has been alluded to, but it has special significance for psychiatrists since, at the moment, they are close to the bottom of the medical professional income market. Another factor, again more intrusive in psychiatry than the other medical disciplines, is the increasing and time-consuming meddling in their clinical practices by governmental and judicial agencies.

As a result, much of the teaching has been relegated to resident house staff and to junior faculty, without providing adequate models for them to emulate and with questionable reward systems. This means that there are fewer teachers with sufficient breadth and general knowledge to deal adequately with the challenge of present day pluralism. The profession, and particularly its younger members, has become so diverse and so fragmented that there are not many capable of understanding and putting into proper perspective the genetic, biological and psychosocial aspects of the behaviour of their patients and their patients' families. Small wonder, then, that students become disappointed in their fragmentary teaching.

Another point is the reduced opportunity open to the student for clinical scholarship. In the past, the fourth year of medical school provided advanced clinical clerkships in all the major clinical disciplines. With the change to an elective fourth year, most students are deprived of the opportunity for sustained, responsible clinical assignments. They have become spectators rather than participant observers of the human condition.

2. In discussing psychoanalytic institutes you speak of 'the narrowness and the arrogance of those who maintain closed systems of belief and practice'. In the next sentence, however, you state: ' ... there is little question that dynamic psychotherapy, as influenced by psychoanalytic psychology, has had a tremendous humanising influence on all of medicine'. How do you reconcile these views?

The political administrative organisation of the American Psychoanalytical Institutes (with the exception noted) is characterised by a narrow system of belief and practice, supported arrogantly by its members. However, as Clemenceau remarked about wars and generals, psychoanalytical psychology was and is too important to be left to practicing psychoanalysts.

Through the medium of several of the academic departments of psychiatry, certain basic notions stemming from psychoanalytical psychology have led to a greater understanding of the doctor–patient relationship (based upon the phenomena of transference and countertransference). It has led to awareness of the universal human experience of anxiety and of regressive behaviour in acute illness, and in the various adaptive and maladaptive devices, including repression and denial, as well as mastery, in responding to chronic illness.

The idea of psychic determinism, the dynamic unconscious mind, and the individual differences between persons due to life experience have been woven into the fabric of general psychology and, for that matter, into common folklore. Psychoanalytical psychology has made possible greater awareness of our affective lives. It has added a significant psychological dimension to the care and treatment of the sick. It has made more understandably human the experiences of our patients and their families.

3. You admit of the possibility that 'there may be no good reason for us to survive as a medical specialty'. What would then happen to psychiatry as we know it?

If the discipline of psychiatry does not offer the challenge and excitement necessary to attract and sustain the interest and attention of young men and women of intelligence and sophistication, it will be replaced by other disciplines which do and can offer the appropriate challenge.

In our real world certain problems remain to be solved; for example, the basic properties of psychotherapy and the enigma of schizophrenia. More broadly and boldly, we have yet to gain understanding of the basic cause or causes of madness.

If psychiatry is to suffer from limited imagination and from restricted resources, workers in psychology, biology, biochemistry and, the social sciences, as well as physicians in disciplines other than psychiatry, will respond to the deficit and pursue new knowledge in manners developed by them.

At the moment a good example is that of behavioural paediatrics which grew, in part, because of the deficit operation of traditional child psychiatry. The latter's negligible contribution to paediatrics led paediatricians, together with psychologists and social scientists, to develop a field which they have called behavioural paediatrics. Its viability is due to its empirical research in maternal–child interaction and in growth and development. More particularly, they have responded to a number of practical needs such as preparing the child and his parents for surgery, concern with the battered and burned child, and further studies of hospital care of children. All of this has been found to be most useful to the paediatrician in his care of the children and families entrusted to him.

Select bibliography

Romano, J. (1950). Basic orientation and education of the medical student. *Journal of the American Medical Association*, **143**, 409–12.
Romano, J. (1961). Teaching of psychiatry to medical students. *Lancet*, ii, 93–5.
Romano, J. (1970). Teaching of psychiatry to medical students: past, present and future. *American Journal of Psychiatry*, **126**, (8), 1115–26.
Romano, J. (1975). Within bareheaded distance, the story of Wing R. (1945–1975). In *To Each His Farthest Star*, ed. J. Romano, chapter 15, pp. 295–318. University of Rochester.
Romano, J. (1977*a*). Requiem or reveille: psychiatry's choice. *Bulletin of the New York Academy of Medicine*, **53**, (9), 787–805.
Romano, J. (1977*b*). Nature of schizophrenia, changes in the observer as well as the observed (1932–1977). *Schizophrenia Bulletin*, **3**, (4), 532–59.
Romano, J. (1979). Chierurgions ought to be wyse, gentyll and sober. *Contemporary Surgery*, **15**, 13–16, 21–3.
Romano, J. (1980). On the teaching of psychiatry to medical students: does it have to get worse before it gets better? *Psychosomatic Medicine*, **42**, 103–11.

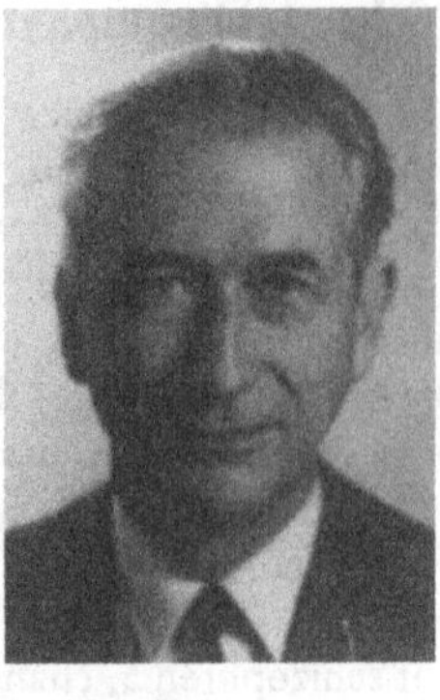

10 · ERIK STROMGREN

Personal background and professional experience

I was born in Copenhagen on 28 November 1909. My parents were Swedes but had spent six years in Germany before they moved to Denmark. They were both active in teaching and research and had many international contacts.

At the age of 14 I became interested in philosophy, psychology and psychiatry. Outstanding local representatives of psychology were Harald Høffding and Alfred Lehmann, whose clear writings impressed me a great deal. I was also fascinated by the psychiatric writings of two of my parents' friends, Alfred Petrén, Professor of Psychiatry at the University of Uppsala, and Axel Herrlin, Professor of Philosophy at the University of Lund.

During my childhood I spent my summer vacations in the home of my mother's sister and her husband, both doctors who were deeply interested in psychiatry. My uncle, Emanuel af Geijerstam, was one of the first practising psychoanalysts in Sweden. I was very much impressed by his devotion to his work with patients. He gave me access to his personal experience and to his unique library (which later on I inherited) containing practically all the published psychoanalytical literature. I think I was 15 when I read Freud's *Uber Psychoanalyse*, which made an enormous impression on me. Shortly afterwards I started reading Eugen Bleuler's *Textbook of Psychiatry*, which has probably influenced me more than any other book on psychiatry. Although I never had the opportunity to meet Bleuler personally I somehow felt very close to his personality which emanates so clearly from his writings. It was with a double satisfaction that later on I acquired the friendship of his son, Manfred Bleuler. For me the attitudes of these two men to psychiatry and to psychiatric patients have been exemplary.

From Eugen Bleuler it was only a short step to Emil Kraepelin and especially Ernst Kretschmer, whose *Körperbau und Charakter* and *Der sensitive Beziehungswahn* I still regard as fundamental contributions to psychiatry. I also read the works of many of Freud's pupils, most of which, however, I found quite disappointing, except for the books by Carl Gustav Jung, Sandor Ferenczi and Otto Rank. At that time there were no trained psychoanalysts in Denmark. There was a growing number of wild analysts who attracted considerable public attention but whose work was inferior. Against this background it was an event when Wilhelm Reich came to Denmark, having emigrated from Germany in 1933. Reich was a gifted lecturer, and his thinking had not begun to assume its later delusional character. Reich spent only a short time in Denmark, and there were no other competent psychoanalysts in the country so that I had no chance to receive psychoanalytical training.

Shortly before finishing my medical studies I had to spend six months in hospital because of a lung infection. This gave me an opportunity to engage in tasks which, in other circumstances, I would probably never have approached. For instance, I started making Rorschach tests on my fellow patients. Rorschach's original book and his collection of plates had been out of print for many years and unavailable in Denmark. Eventually, a new edition was printed which gave me the possibility of applying this technique, probably for the first time in Denmark. My co-patients were, of course, readily available as subjects.

Next, I started some enquiries among the patients in order to acquire knowledge about a selection of mentally normal persons concerning the structure of their personalities, especially of their self-images and their levels of aspiration. I usually started these interviews by means of an abrupt question: 'What is your goal in life?' It was fascinating to experience how unprepared the interviewees were to answer this question. They all became very engaged in the discussion of the problem, and their responses clearly demonstrated the existence of important ingredients in their self-image of which they were normally quite unaware. On the basis of these results I developed a description of the self-image (*Persönlichkeitsbewusstsein*) and expressed the viewpoint that psychogenic delusions arise when the subject comes into a situation in which it is necessary to make a sudden radical revision of the self-image in a negative direction.

The start of a case of *sensitiver Beziehungswahn* is a clear example of such mechanisms.

During my stay in hospital I had the opportunity to read extensively, but even then so much was being published on psychiatry that it was impossible to read it all. I formed the opinion that through selective reading important topics and findings might be overlooked and that there was a danger of ignoring material which, for some reason, did not appeal to me. I therefore undertook the task of reading a journal volume of 800 pages, page by page, in which I encountered several articles which ordinarily I would certainly have avoided but which turned out to be very interesting. Among them was an excellent paper on diffuse sclerosis, or leucoencephalopathy as it is now usually called. I became deeply interested in disorders belonging to this group and this later led to cooperation with the neuropathologist Axel V. Neel, and the anatomy professor, Lárus Einarson, with whom I jointly investigated a number of families in which diffuse sclerosis was prevalent.

I graduated in 1934, but during the preceding years I had been working for several periods in a psychiatric hospital (Vordingborg), the head of which was Hjalmar Helweg, later to become Professor of Psychiatry at the University of Copenhagen. After graduation I worked again in the same hospital, an experience of decisive importance for me. Helweg was a man with outstanding qualities, a highly intelligent, learned and kind person with an accurate knowledge of each of his 800 patients. I have always felt since that with mental patients one of the most important things one can do for them, in nearly all cases, is to *know* them and to be able to distinguish them from all other human beings. A psychiatric diagnosis may be a severe obstacle to the acquirement of this goal.

My work at the Vordingborg Hospital gave me a first contact with people coming from the island of Bornholm, which belonged to the catchment area of the hospital. It struck me that it would be especially easy to carry out epidemiological and genetic studies on that island. The local dialect is extremely characteristic and diagnosable even in its mildest forms; in addition, a number of names are characteristic of indigenous families. Before my graduation I had already decided to conduct an epidemiological study on the island. During a vacation there I made a number of home visits and found the population to be most cooperative and sympathetic towards research. I obtained an appointment at the local general hospital, and over the following years I collected the material which became the basis for my doctoral thesis. The field work included about 1,000 home visits. Although my principal aim was to do research,

I now think that other facets of this work came to assume still more importance for me. During the time I spent on Bornholm I came to know practically all those individuals with any mental abnormality, of whom only a small fraction had ever been admitted to a psychiatric hospital or been in contact with psychiatry in other ways. The existence of this large number of undiagnosed and mostly untreated mentally disordered human beings seemed to me to constitute one of the most important problems of psychiatry.

In those pre-war years an interest in psychiatric epidemiology was unusual in Scandinavia. In 1935 I therefore visited the Deutsche Forschungsanstalt für Psychiatrie in Munich which was at that time the centre in which epidemiological methodology was most advanced. Several of the figures who were to become prominent in the field of psychiatric genetics and epidemiology visited this institution in those years, for instance Eliot Slater, Erik Essen-Möller and Franz Kallmann. My closest contact was Bruno Schulz, a unique personality whose conscientiousness in research together with his complete honesty made it quite impossible for the political forces at that time to influence his research in any way.

From Bornholm I moved to Copenhagen, where I obtained an appointment at the Department of Psychiatry of the University of Copenhagen. This newly established department was headed by Professor August Wimmer, the most learned psychiatrist whom I have ever met. In addition, he was a most competent neurologist, as demonstrated by his monographs on epidemic encephalitis. Wimmer's interests covered all branches of psychiatry. Of special importance for Scandinavian psychiatry is his monograph on psychogenic psychoses (1916). This monograph, unfortunately never translated into any other language, was founded on a convincing collection of case histories. It opened the eyes of all Scandinavian psychiatrists to the importance of this group of disorders.

In between my duties at the psychiatric clinic I had some appointments in somatic departments. In 1943 I moved to Aarhus to take up a newly established post as Reader in Psychiatry. The University of Aarhus, founded in 1928, was gradually building a medical school and the time had come for a course in psychiatry to be established. The clinical base for this teaching was the local mental hospital, situated in the suburb of Risskov. In 1945 the superintendent of the hospital, Aage Thune Jacobsen, retired and I became his successor. At the same time I was appointed to the chair of psychiatry, and it became clear that in connection with this new university there would be unique opportunities for creating a psychiatric teaching and research institution.

The mental hospital at Risskov is a regional hospital, the only psychiatric institution in the area, taking care of all types of mental disorders with the exception of the mentally retarded who, in Denmark, are traditionally treated in separate institutions. The hospital is located near a large city and could therefore serve as a natural centre for outpatient facilities. Whereas the work was gratifying in Vordingborg, a similar institution, I had been disappointed by the organisation of psychiatry in the city of Copenhagen, where all acute cases were admitted to the psychiatric wards of the general hospitals. There they could be treated for only a few weeks, and had to be transferred to the municipal psychiatric hospital if they needed longer inpatient care. To me the ideal institution was the "complete" psychiatric hospital, located in the middle of the area served by the hospital.

At Risskov I felt that a truly comprehensive psychiatry of this type could be realised. The attachment to the university provided special obligations with regard to a complete coverage of function, and for teaching and research it was necessary for all kinds of psychiatric facilities to be available and all subspecialties of psychiatry to be represented. Fortunately, the attitude of the administrative authorities was very favourable to these ideas. At that time the hospital, like most psychiatric hospitals in Denmark, was a state hospital, governed by a department of the Ministry of Interior Affairs. This department gave full support to the development of the new activities and facilities in the hospital. There was excellent cooperation with the university which, although formally private, was financed mainly by the state. This arrangement represented an administrative advance, since there could be no disagreement between university and hospital with regard to the payment for those activities which were created for the purpose of teaching and research.

During the war and the immediate post-war years the financial situation was strained. It was not possible to construct new buildings for the new activities, which had to be improvised in existing buildings, in attics and basements and in staff apartments. During the 1950s and 1960s the situation improved rapidly and a number of different departments were created. The order in which they came into existence depended mainly on the availability of qualified leaders. First came a neuropathological laboratory; later, a biochemical laboratory, which developed into an institute of biological psychiatry, including psychopharmacology, and a cytogenetic laboratory. Alongside these establishments a number of specialised clinical departments were developed: the outpatient clinic with satellites in a number of towns within the catchment area, a clinic for outpatient treatment of neuroses, a clinic for alcoholics, a department for forensic psychiatry and a department for clinical psychology.

The necessary training facilities for dynamic psychotherapy took some time to become established in Denmark. Personally, I had intended to obtain a regular training in dynamic psychotherapy but in the pre-war years and during the war this was not feasible in Denmark. When, after the war, possibilities for training in other countries became available, I had reached a senior academic position and found it more useful to help young psychiatrists to have such a training than to go through it myself. The first to go to the United States for regular psychoanalytical training was Poul Faergeman, who had just finished his psychiatric education and had published his large thesis on psychogenic psychoses. This study consisted of a follow-up of all cases of psychogenic psychoses which had been admitted to August Wimmer's clinic in Copenhagen between 1924 and 1926 and had been re-investigated after 15 to 20 years. Later, when Faergeman had been working as an analyst in the United States for a number of years, he wrote a new English edition of his monograph which was influenced by his analytical experience.

Faergeman had intended to return to Denmark and start a school of dynamic psychiatry, but since he remained for 12 years in the United States his place was taken by Thorkil Vanggaard. Other associates who worked abroad were Harry Stokholm, who studied dynamic psychiatry in Boston, and Villars Lunn, who studied clinical psychology at the Maudsley Hospital. It was fortunate that over the years the staff of the Risskov Hospital was supplemented by a number of highly qualified psychotherapists, thus creating excellent possibilities for psychotherapeutic training locally.

With the advent of efficient somatic therapies during the 1950s a new situation arose. The prospects for providing effective treatment to a much larger number of psychiatric patients improved radically. It was challenging to learn from epidemiological studies of the existence of a large number of patients who had never been in contact with psychiatry but who would now be accessible to treatment. For me personally it was especially tempting to try to use my knowledge of the population in Bornholm to initiate a comprehensive community psychiatry programme there. Unfortunately, this was impracticable since Bornholm did not belong to the catchment area of the Risskov Hospital and, furthermore, was located farther away from Risskov than any other part of the country. Instead, a project was started with the population of the island of Samsø which belongs to the catchment area of the hospital. The goal of this study was to ascertain all individuals on the island who were in need of psychiatric treatment and to offer them optimal therapeutic opportunities. This work was started in 1957 in close cooperation with the general practitioners of the island. The work was made possible by a grant from the Ford Foundation, which gave the staff excellent facilities for a period of five years, after which the Danish state took over the financing of the project.

When the Samsø project had been in progress for a few years, a reasonably accurate knowledge of the psychiatric needs of that population was obtained. Since the population could be regarded as representative of the Danish rural population, some generalisations could be made, not only with regard to the frequencies of different kinds of mental disorder, but also with regard to the nature and extent of facilities necessary for adequate diagnosis and treatment and, where possible, prevention.

The Samsø project was part of an epidemiological programme which came to serve as a basis for the establishment of the so-called Institute of Psychiatric Demography in 1967. This Institute comprises also the National Psychiatric Register, which receives information concerning all admissions to and discharges from psychiatric institutions in Denmark and which, therefore, in cooperation with the National Health Service, assumes responsibility for the statistics and annual reports of these institutions. In addition, these statistics serve as the basis for the planning of mental health services in Denmark.

In 1976 the organisation of mental health services underwent a complete change. Until then the mental hospitals had been administered mainly by the state, but thenceforward the counties assumed responsibility for them. It became necessary to discover the adequate amount of psychiatric facilities for each county, a difficult question since the demand for psychiatric services had been changing rapidly. Among psychiatrists opinions were divided concerning the merits of developing psychiatric units in general hospitals compared with exclusively psychiatric institutions. During the last decade, however, opinions have converged. In 1970 the Danish Psychiatric Association published a comprehensive report concerning the future development of psychiatry. It stated that the smallest units which could function independently must have at least 60 beds and, in addition, it was recommended that, wherever possible, a number of such units should be built together, for instance in groups of three to six units. In several places where small units of 20 to 30 beds already exist it is planned to expand them to a size which can allow them to function as a complete hospital.

Current status of psychiatry

To describe the present status of psychiatry is not easy since general agreement is lacking. Concepts and fashions are accepted, rejected and combined in a variety of ways. During the 1940s and 1950s, for example, genetic concepts were out of favour with American psychiatrists, who were then wedded to psychoanalysis. In the Soviet Union, by contrast, psychoanalysis was virtually non-existent. In the Scandinavian countries opinions were divided, but one characteristic figure emerged: the bearded workers in the mental health field who detested genetics, preached psychoanalysis, and declared an allegiance to communism.

That period of maximal divergence with regard to basic viewpoints has fortunately passed. It is encouraging to see that the different factions within psychiatry are becoming more tolerant of each other. Everywhere rapid changes are in progress. It is, however, possible to describe current trends which in Denmark resemble those which are to be found elsewhere in the Western World. Some generalisations are therefore permissible.

There is a general trend towards the expansion of outpatient services. In Denmark, where traditionally there have been very few hospital beds, their numbers will probably not be reduced very much: an increasing fraction of the manpower in the hospitals is likely to be directed towards outpatient work of the community mental health type.

Within the hospitals the scene has changed radically during the last few decades. Since 1957 census studies of all psychiatric hospitals have been conducted every five years. The total number of beds is unchanged, but the diagnostic and age distributions have changed considerably. The dominant trend is a reduction of the prevalence rates for schizophrenia and an increase in the rate for geriatric disorders. Before World War II 75 per cent of all schizophrenics were in institutions; today only 25 per cent are inpatients. This change is especially marked for female schizophrenics.

The increasing number of geriatric patients is causing a great problem for the hospitals, which are compelled to accept disturbed old patients but are very often unable to discharge them again even if their condition has improved sufficiently. Many wards are filled with patients who need not be in hospital but could as well be treated in homes for the elderly or in nursing homes. Financial and administrative reasons prevent them from entering appropriate institutions. In Denmark, for example, the county pays for them as long as they remain in hospital; when they are in a nursing home the municipalities have to pay 50 per cent of the costs so that, not surprisingly, they are reluctant to provide the necessary number of nursing homes.

This is simply one example of how artificial administrative barriers impede the rational use of existing facilities. Such obstacles are increasing in number in an era of decentralisation. The care of chronic mental patients is further complicated by the fact that the building and staffing standards of modern nursing homes are often higher than those prevailing in old psychiatric hospitals, where the cost per patient day may be lower than in a modern nursing home. It is therefore tempting for society to let patients stay where their maintenance is cheapest. The cost per patient day in a modern nursing home has now become so high that it is questionable whether the taxpayers will agree to an expansion of this sector. The only solution would seem to be the return of a considerable fraction of the patients in care to their families or to some kind of family care, supervised and supported by home-visiting nurses and other professional supervisors.

The composition of the staffs of psychiatric institutions has changed radically. A generation ago the personnel consisted mainly of a small group of doctors who administered the work of a large nursing staff in an authoritative manner. Recently, the nursing staff has taken a more responsible part in the work, and new professions with increasing responsibilities are represented on the staff, including social work, clinical psychology and occupational therapy. Simultaneously, the position of the physicians has declined despite the increasing numbers of doctors in psychiatric institutions. Their administrative responsibilities have been partly distributed elsewhere, and what is left has been divided among other mental health professionals who believe that the competence of psychiatrists within the psychiatric field is limited and does not warrant their leading position. Most members of these parapsychiatric professions feel that the more important etiological factors in psychiatry are of a psychological nature and that treatment should be modified accordingly, leaving only a very small field for the doctors' special competence. Although this is to some degree an expression of wishful thinking among the members of new and expanding professions, there is an understandable basis for the lack of confidence in the value of the medical contribution to psychiatry. It cannot be denied that in many places and periods psychiatry has not attracted the *élite* of the medical profession, and that there have been times when it was too easy to acquire senior psychiatric positions without adequate competence. Further, a heavy work load often prevents psychiatrists from keeping up with developments in their speciality.

On the other hand, it cannot be claimed that most members of the new professions have any greater competence. They have been trained for particular aspects of psychiatry but not for evaluating and treating mental disorders as a whole. Almost all those who are working within the field of psychiatry, whether medically qualified or not, feel that what can be accomplished in the treatment of many patients is unsatisfactory. Some, including most psychiatrists, feel that psychiatry is an extremely complex and difficult discipline which has still to mature. Others feel that it is only 'traditional' treatments which are misplaced, and that 'alternative' therapies would change everything for the better. Yet, despite a sometimes semi-religious conviction concerning the etiology and treatment of psychiatric disorders, the non-psychiatrists also seem to feel an urgent need for more knowledge. Such groups attend a great number of postgraduate courses, symposia and other meetings, which, in combination with the reduction of the number of working hours of all staff-members, has the effect of diminishing the time devoted to patient care. Nevertheless, the prospects are perhaps not as bad as one might fear. There are signs that an increasing number of psychiatric staff-members feel uncomfortable about their distance from their patients and want to re-establish a more direct and realistic contact with them.

So much for anti-psychiatry *within* psychiatry. At the same time the anti-psychiatric movement *outside* psychiatry should not be forgotten because of its potential influence on public opinion. Even if mature politicians and administrators can see that much of the anti-psychiatric talk is ill-founded, they may use clichés as excuses for not giving sufficient support to existing psychiatric facilities.

Future prospects of psychiatry

It can be anticipated that the changing trends in the composition of patient groups in hospitals will continue, especially the decrease of schizophrenia and the increase of geriatric disorders. Yet, although an increasing part of psychiatric work will be directed towards the community, it is obvious that mental illness is widespread and that it is utopian to aim at the provision of universal psychiatric care by psychiatric specialists. Most mentally ill patients sooner or later come into contact with general practitioners who should be better placed to treat these patients, though they often feel that the appropriate treatment lies beyond their sphere of competence. It is therefore necessary that practitioners should receive training which makes it possible for them to encounter these patients with knowledge and confidence. The post-graduate psychiatric training of general practitioners has, until now, been mostly of limited relevance to this task. It would be of great value if the practitioners, often working in group practices, could have regular contact with a visiting psychiatrist with whom they could discuss their psychiatric cases and obtain specialised advice concerning examination and treatment. In some cases admission to hospital or referral to a specialist would be necessary; in the great majority of cases, however, the practitioner should be able to carry on the treatment supervised by the psychiatrist.

In making predictions about future developments I find it challenging to recall the predictions I would have made a generation ago and to ascertain to what degree these have been confirmed or refuted. With regard to schizophrenia, for example, I had not anticipated that the treatment of this disease would become radically more effective. I was convinced that schizophrenia was predominantly genetically determined, attributing only some 20–30 per cent of the causation to environmental factors which were, however, largely unknown. According to this contention, the genes could be supposed to lead to some metabolic disorder which in turn induced the primary, relatively immutable, symptoms. The primary symptoms would cause changes in the personality of the patient and in the patient's relationship to the surroundings, inducing secondary, psychological reactions which were partly understandable. These secondary, psychogenic symptoms might even be responsible for the major part of the symptomatology. No wonder, therefore, that psychological factors could occasionally modify the symptomatology radically from one hour to the next. At the same time, experience with intensive environmental therapy, although occasionally encouraging, has, in general, not been so rewarding that major progress is to be expected in the near future. Against this background the often striking improvements associated with pharmacotherapy in combination with rehabilitation measures are impressive. On the other hand, these changes are not qualitatively different from what could be anticipated from the above-mentioned theory concerning the aetiology of schizophrenia. It was not so much the therapeutic successes as the results of genetic studies which showed beyond doubt that the environmental forces played a greater role in the pathogenesis of schizophrenia than had been supposed before. We seem, however, to be left with the same uncertainty concerning the nature of these environmental factors. It thus seems impossible to make any predictions concerning etiological research in schizophrenia, whereas it seems probable that therapy will continue to improve.

With regard to manic-depressive disorder, clinical experience has taught me that the concept should be wider than I had believed earlier. Refined clinical observations, in combination with genetic studies and the effects of modern therapies, seem to indicate that there are many atypical affective states which belong somehow to a common group of mood disorders, whose most clear-cut form is the classical manic-depressive illness. Attempts to make distinctions within this group, for instance by contrasting monopolar and bipolar forms, have never appealed to me. I have always regarded the basis of manic-depressive disorder to be of a mainly physical nature, environmental factors playing only a limited role in a small number of cases. That somatic therapies have brought about the first real advances in the management of this disorder is therefore not surprising. I cannot see that contemporary metabolic investigations, however technically developed, have brought us essential new knowledge concerning aetiology and pathogenesis, but I have no doubt that the solution will come through investigations of this nature. With regard to research on manic-depressive disorder we seem to be especially well placed: the fact that the disorder can be kept under control by means of an agent as simple as the lithium ion seems to present opportunities which are not apparent with any other psychiatric condition. At present the most serious obstacle to the optimal treatment of manic-depressives is the anti-medical attitude which is now so widespread, even among many who have responsibility for the fate of the manic-depressives.

One of the major disappointments has been concerned with the efficacy of psychotherapy. This has improved, but not nearly as much as I had anticipated. Progress in psychotherapy should be measured not only by improvement of the patient's condition, but also by the *time* it has taken to obtain improvement. In the beginning of the psychoanalytical era, when most analysts treated patients by means of orthodox techniques for many years, psychoanalysis was a completely asocial therapy. To me, the most important task of psychotherapists is to develop methods which demand so little time that the majority of those in need of such treatment can obtain it. At present it seems to me that research in this field is much more important than the application of therapy.

I had not anticipated the youth rebellion. In retrospect it is, however, not so surprising to find a natural, innate antagonism between generations. At the turn of the century parents still decided what their children should do and where they should live. This era of authority became a principal target for attack. When personal freedom in a social sense had been obtained, the children were still economically dependent on the parents. Having obtained relative economic independence, the young still felt repressed by the parental generation's restrictive pressure on them in sexual matters. Sexual liberation having been obtained, the welfare society, with its ideals of material security, became an obvious target.

Although the youth rebellion may fade away, this is less likely to be the case with the problems of drug addiction. As the object of strong financial interests, it will probably continue and remain one of psychiatry's greatest concerns, although probably it will be increasingly superseded by the dramatic rise in the consumption of alcohol.

Nor had I anticipated the rise of anti-psychiatry. I could not have predicted that eventually psychiatry would be regarded by many as one of the main evils of humanity, with psychiatrists in the role of the malignant tools of ruthless capitalistic forces. By contrast, in my younger days my main concern about the public was its disinterest in psychiatry or, even worse, its active misinterpretations, disclosing a widespread conviction about mental disorder as a chronic condition unamenable to treatment. At first anti-psychiatry seemed, at least, to have the merit of stimulating more active interest in psychiatry. Everyone working in psychiatry was fully aware of its drawbacks and could only be glad that people outside the field of psychiatry were obviously becoming more involved. It was disappointing to see that, instead of criticising the real deficiencies, anti-psychiatrists preferred to attack windmills. With the aid of mass media and certain political forces it became all too easy for them to turn public opinion against the existing psychiatric services.

Future developments on this front are difficult to predict. In some countries the anti-psychiatric wave has already receded; in others it is still fluctuating. Anti-psychiatry is certainly no new trend; on the contrary, it is immanent in the development of psychiatry. In Denmark 100 years ago there was a very active public anti-psychiatric movement. The main victim of attacks at that time was Professor Knud Pontoppidan, head of the University Psychiatric Clinic, who eventually wrote a book on his experiences during the attacks on him. The books ends with a sigh of resignation: 'Even if I may not profit myself from my public intervention, it could possibly be of some help to the next victim when sometime the tide will bring back a new wave of anti-psychiatry.' Anti-psychiatry has brought some good and more harm. But even if the balance-sheet is negative, it should not be discouraging for those who carry the responsibility for the treatment of the mentally ill. The daily experience of the radical changes towards the betterment of the fate of the mentally disordered following the advances of therapy during the last decades should lead to the view of anti-psychiatry as no more than a minor nuisance.

Questions and answers

1. Concerning psychotherapy (p. 163) you state that 'research in this field is much more important than the application of therapy'. What type of research have you in mind?

It is, of course, extremely difficult to design a research project which could demonstrate differences in the efficacy of different kinds of psychotherapy compared with somatic treatment or no treatment. In view of the fact that any kind of psychotherapy will need rather a long time to become effective, it is ethically impossible to employ a control group or a placebo group which would be without any kind of treatment for a long period. Nor does it seem possible to select a large group of clinically similar cases and then allocate sub-groups to different kinds of psychotherapy. It is not possible to compel a therapist to employ a type of therapy which he does not regard as appropriate for a particular patient.

I think the only thing which can be done is to organise large-scale cooperation between a great number of psychotherapists who should agree on the criteria for degrees of symptoms and incapacity as well as criteria of improvement. Before the commencement of treatment each patient should be assessed by a small group of therapists who would agree on the description of the patient's status. After a certain time the same group should reassess the patient, trying to evaluate the impact of treatment.

This would be a procedure which cannot in any way compete with procedures applicable to somatic therapeutic trials. It would demand much in the way of manpower, it would be very costly and it would take many years to collect a sufficiently large group of patients. There would be many drop-outs and many changes of therapy, and other factors would diminish the material. On the other hand, it does not seem ethically defensible to continue blindly with psychotherapy in the hope that it may be of some use. If really convinced that psychotherapy helps, it is ethically justifiable to apply it. It is, however, also an indispensable duty to convince those who are paying for psychotherapy. There will always be the risk that one day they will refuse to pay until some kind of proof that psychotherapy is useful has been established. Therefore, it would be unethical to abstain from attempts at carrying out such research.

2. In discussing the future prospects of psychiatry you make little mention of the potential contribution of the basic sciences. How would you assess their place in the development of the subject?

Concerning the endogenous psychoses, I mention that in the aetiology of schizophrenia biological factors must play a considerable role, in the aetiology of manic-depressive disorder a dominant role. It is obvious that the basic sciences have a crucial role in the exploration of these aetiological factors. In schizophrenia the biological part of the aetiology *may* be relatively homogenous and therefore reasonably accessible to research, whereas the environmental factors are probably most heterogenous and therefore much more difficult to identify. Even with regard to neuroses and reactive psychoses which have a predominantly psychogenic aetiology there is, in most cases, some kind of a predisposition, a special vulnerability, which may be connected with anomalies in certain receptor functions in the brain. Biological research is therefore also indicated in these cases.

3. How do you now regard the concept of the psychogenic psychosis which, as you mentioned, has played a special role in the thinking of Scandinavian psychiatrists?

The concept of psychogenic or reactive psychogenic psychosis has been in constant use in the Scandinavian countries since the beginning of the century. In Denmark about 10 per cent of all admissions to psychiatric institutions carry this diagnosis, i.e. about 20 per cent of all psychoses. It is therefore incomprehensible to Scandinavian psychiatrists that the glossary of the International Classification of Diseases (9th edition) still regards these cases as 'rare'. It should not be forgotten that Scandinavians are not the only psychiatrists who feel that this concept is necessary. In French-speaking, Russian, Japanese and many other countries, especially in Asia and Africa, reactive psychoses also constitute an important group of mental disorders. It is therefore important that the World Health Organisation has recently started an international collaborative study on these 'acute psychoses'.

References

Bleuler, E. (1923). *Lehrbuch der Psychiatrie* (vierte Auflage). Berlin: Verlag von Julius Springer.

Danish Psychiatric Association Report (1970) Betaenkning om psykiatriens udvikling i Danmark i den naermeste fremtid. *Fra Sundhedsstyrelsen*, 5, 225–46.

Faergeman, P. M. (1945). *De psykogene psykoser belyst gennem katamnestiske undersøgelser*. København: Munksgaard. 425pp.

Faergeman, P. M. (1963). *Psychogenic Psychoses. A Description and Follow-up of Psychoses following Psychological Stress*. London: Butterworth. 268pp.

Freud, S. (1910). *Uber Psychoanalyse.* Fünf Vorlesungen gehalten zur zwanzigjährigen Gründungsfeier der Clark University in Worcester, Mass., September 1909. Leipzig, Vienna: Deuticke. 62pp.

Kretschmer, E. (1918). *Der sensitive Beziehungswahn.* Berlin: Verlag von Julius Springer. 166pp.

Kretschmer, E. (1921). *Körperbau und Charakter.* Berlin: Verlag von Julius Springer. 192pp.

Pontoppidan, K. (1897). *6te Afdelings Jammersminde.* København: Th. Linds Efterfølger. 48pp.

Wimmer, A. (1916). Psykogene Sindssygdomsformer. In *St. Hans Hospital 1816–1916.* Jubilaeumsskrift, pp. 85–216. København: G. E. C. Gads Forlag. (Reprinted in 1980 by Janssenpharma.)

Select bibliography

Strömgren, E. (1935). Zum Ersatz des Weinbergschen "abgekürzten Verfahrens". Zugleich ein Beitrag zur Frage von der Erblichkeit des Erkrankungsalters bei der Schizophrenie. (A substitute for Weinberg's 'abridged method.' With a contribution to the question of inheritance of age of onset in schizophrenia.) *Z. ges. Neurol. Psychiat.*, 153, 784–97.

Strömgren, E. (1937). Uber anthropometrische Indices zur Unterscheidung von Körperbautypen. (On anthropometric indices for Distinction of body types.) *Z. ges. Neurol. Psychiat.*, 159, 75–81.

Strömgren, E. (1938). Contributions à la méthode typologique en psychiatrie. (Contributions to the typological method in psychiatry.) *Biotypologie*, 6, 1–16.

Strömgren, E. (1938). *Beiträge zur psychiatrischen Erblehre.* Auf Grund von Untersuchungen an einer Inselbevölkerung. (*Contributions to Psychiatric Genetics based on investigations of an Island population.*) København: Munksgaard. 258pp.

Strömgren, E. (1940). *Episodiske Psykoser.* Fem Forelæsninger. (Episodic Psychoses.) København: Munksgaard. 131pp.

Einarson, L., Neel, A. V. & Strömgren, E. (1944). On the problem of diffuse brain sclerosis with special reference to the familial forms (Leukoencephalopathia diffusa progressiva hereditaria). *Acta Jutlandica*, 16, 1. 178pp.

Hermann, K. & Strömgren, E. (1944). Paroxysmal disturbances of consciousness in verified localized brain affections. With special regard to the so-called "dreamy states". *Acta Psychiat. (Kbh)*, 19, 175–94.

Strömgren, E. (1945). *Om Bevidsthedsforstyrrelser.* (Disorders of consciousness.) København: Munksgaard. 72pp.

Strömgren, E. (1946). Mental sequelae of suicidal attempts by hanging. *Acta Psychiat. (Kbh.)*, 21, 753–80.

Strömgren, E. (1950). Statistical and genetical population studies within psychiatry. Methods and principal results. In: *Congrès international de psychiatrie, Paris 1950*, pp. 155–92, + Discussion. Paris: Hermann & Cie.

Schou, M., Juel-Nielsen, N., Voldby, H. & Strömgren, E. (1954). The treatment of manic psychoses by the administration of lithium salts. *J. Neurol. Neurosurg. Psychiat.*, **17**, 250–7.

Strömgren, E. (1955). Psykiatriske problemer i almindelig lægepraksis. Resultater af en statistisk undersøgelse. (Psychiatric problems in general practice. Results of a statistical investigation.) *Ugeskr. Læg.*, **117**, 230–2.

Welner, J. & Strömgren, E. (1958). Clinical and genetic studies on benign schizophreniform psychoses based on a follow-up. *Acta Psychiat. Scand.*, **33**, 377–99.

Strömgren, E. (1958). Pathogenese der verschiedenen Formen von psychogenen Psychosen. (Pathogenesis of the different types of psychogenic psychoses.) In: *Mehrdimensionale Diagnostik und Therapie*. Festschrift zum 70. Geburtstag von Herrn Professor Dr. med. Dr. phil. h.c. Ernst Kretschmer, pp. 67–70. Stuttgart: Georg Thieme Verlag.

Strömgren, E. (1958). Mental health service planning in Denmark. *Dan. Med. Bull.*, 5, 1–47.

Arentsen, K. & Strömgren, E. (1959). Patients in Danish psychiatric hospitals. Results of a census in 1957. *Acta Jutlandica*, **31**, 1. 49pp. + Appendix.

Einarson, L. & Strömgren, E. (1961). Diffuse progressive leucoencephalopathy (diffuse cerebral sclerosis) and its relationship to amaurotic idiocy. *Acta Jutlandica*, **33**, 1. 84pp.

Juel-Nielsen, N. & Strömgren, E. (1963). Five years later. A comparison between census studies of patients in psychiatric institutions in Denmark in 1957 and 1962. *Acta Jutlandica*, **35**, 1. 44pp. + Appendix.

Strömgren, E. (1963). The psychiatric hospital as centre of community psychiatry. *Comprehens. Psychiat.*, **4**, 433–41.

Strömgren, E. (1967). Psychiatrische Genetik. (Psychiatric genetics.) In *Psychiatrie der Gegenwart*, ed. H. W. Gruhle, R. Jung, W. Mayer-Gross & M. Müller, 1/1A, pp. 1–59. Berlin, Heidelberg and New York: Springer Verlag.

Strömgren, E. (1968). Contributions to psychiatric epidemiology and genetics. *Acta Jutlandica* **40**. 86pp.

Juel-Nielsen N. & Strömgren, E. (1969). Ten years later. A comparison between census studies of patients in psychiatric institutions in Denmark in 1957, 1962 and 1967. *Acta Jutlandica*, **41**, 2.

Strömgren, E., Dalby, A., Dalby, M. A. & Ranheim, B. (1970). Cataract, deafness, cerebellar ataxia, psychosis and dementia – a new syndrome. *Acta Neurol. Scand.*, suppl. **43**, 261–2.

McCabe, M. S. & Strömgren, E. (1975). Reactive psychoses. A family study. *Arch. Gen. Psychiat.*, **32**, 447–54.

Strömgren, E. (1975). Genetic factors in the origin of schizophrenia. In *On the Origin of Schizophrenic Psychoses*, ed. H. M. van Praag (Symposium organised by the Interdisciplinary Society of Biological Psychiatry), pp. 7–18. Amsterdam: De Erven Bohn BV.

Weeke, A. & Strömgren, E. (1978). Fifteen years later. A comparison of patients in Danish psychiatric institutions in 1957, 1962, 1967 and 1972. *Acta Psychiat. Scand.*, 57, 129–44.

Strömgren, E., Kyst, E., Ryberg, I. & Weeke, A. (1979). Estimation of need on the basis of field survey findings. In: *Estimating Needs for Mental Health Care. A Contribution of Epidemiology*, ed. H. Häfner, pp. 37–42. Berlin, Heidelberg and New York: Springer-Verlag.

Strömgren, E. (1979). *Psykiatri* (13. udgave). (*Psychiatry*, 13th edition.) København: Munksgaard.

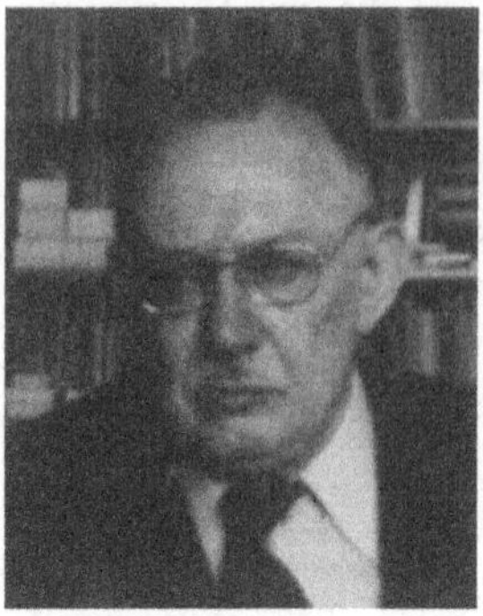

11 · HANS STROTZKA

Personal background and professional experience

As a psychoanalyst I am convinced that early childhood experiences are the main source of later traits and trends in the personality. There seems to me to be overwhelming clinical evidence for this hypothesis if one has learned to look closely enough at mental development. Despite this fundamental tenet, the biographical introduction to this chapter will be short, simply because it seems to me sufficient for the understanding of later events to make public only the main lines of my development. Some degree of privacy is a human right and I find the demand for total revelation, which is nowadays so strongly urged, rather dubious.

I was born in Vienna in 1917, the second child of a middle-class family. My father was a civil servant in the personnel department of the central post-office, a quiet, rather liberal person with some creative talent, especially in the spheres of painting and small handicraft. My mother, a former teacher, later became totally devoted to her household. I remember her mainly standing at her coal-heated stove and cooking for hours on end. She was a Roman Catholic but her religious views were not extreme. In the first 10 years of my life we lived in a two-room flat at Klosterneuburg, a small town 12 kilometres upstream from Vienna, dominated by a large monastery and a cathedral. Without a bathroom, we took our weekly bath in a small zinc bath-tub in the kitchen.

The most vivid experience of my early life was certainly a strong oral deprivation, resulting from hunger and detected by our general practitioner. After some extra nutrition from official and private sources this was soon corrected, but basic oral character traits have remained through my life: a strong tendency to eat, drink and smoke, a general friendly extraversion, and a slight latent aggression, manifested mainly by a certain kind of humour which seems to be difficult for others to understand. In psychoanalytical terms a depressive defence is apparent. The second strong influence was a savage competition with my sister, who is five years older than me. She was always the best in her class and I developed an enormous drive to reach her level of maturity and intellectual competence. Both these factors, allied to the unavoidable oedipal constellation, are probably the roots of a highly developed curiosity which may be my main character trait. From my early years I became a great reader, with a very broad scope of interests.

When I was 12 years old, we moved to a house of our own. Having a room to myself with a view of green trees made me very happy. In school I was always the best or one of the best pupils without any great effort on my part, but I was rather poor at sports and handicraft.

Growing up in Austria's first republic was to be exposed to dangerous political passions. A national youth movement gained an influence on me and it took me years to distance myself from it. Years of analysis were later necessary to work through this narcissistic frustration at having been stupid enough to have been so profoundly deceived.

I would have liked to study philology but our family doctor persuaded me to study medicine as the safest career in uncertain times. From the beginning I was interested in psychotherapy and joined a student association for medical psychology where the courses included those devoted to psychoanalysis by Erwin Stengel.

Six months after my graduation in 1940 I was called up to the army. During the following six years I served chiefly in neuro-psychiatric wards because I was lucky enough to have worked for six months in the Neuro-psychiatric University Clinic in Vienna before my military service. Another fortunate event was a severe injury at the beginning of the Russian war which lowered my level of medical fitness. Having worked mainly in neurology before, I made my first contacts with foreign literature in psychiatry as an American prisoner-of-war in Italy.

In 1942 I married Veronika Bartl. Our two sons were born in 1942 and 1944 and we now have three grandchildren. After the war I worked from 1946 to 1951 in a dominantly neurological hospital, but one which included 'minor' psychiatry under Erwin Stransky and later Hans Hoff. In 1948 I spent six months at a large mental hospital. From 1951 to

1971 I worked as head of a psychotherapeutic outpatient clinic of the compulsory health-insurance scheme for workers. During this time I became, in 1959–60, the Mental Health Adviser of the UNHCR in Geneva on the basis of my previous mental health work with Hungarian refugees between 1956 and 1958. At that time we organised the camp-clearance programme for displaced persons in Germany, Austria, Italy and Greece.

In addition, I acquired some experience in an outpatient clinic for epileptic children, as a teacher in psychiatry at a social-work school, as a psychiatrist in a child-guidance clinic for adolescents and finally in town and country planning.

My training in the Vienna Psychoanalytic Association lasted from 1950 to 1958. Before then I had participated in Igor Caruso's working group for depth psychology from 1948 to 1949. Since 1968 I have been a teaching analyst. Principally as an autodidact I have received some experience in autogenic training, hypnosis, group and family therapy and, above all, in psychoanalytical oriented psychotherapy. In 1971 I became Director of the newly founded Institute of Depth Psychology and Psychotherapy of the University of Vienna, and I have based its activities on the foundations of methodological pluralism and interdisciplinary activity.

So far I have tried to outline a skeleton to a life curriculum, necessarily simplified and sketchy. To put even a little flesh to the bones is not easy, as I am unable to say that I was fortunate enough to develop any identifiable school of thought.

As an undergraduate I was a 'demonstrator' (a kind of tutor) in physiology and pathology and I was selected for a scholarship in neurophysiology with Muralt in Bern. The war prevented these plans from maturing. The half year at the Vienna clinic with Pötzl was much too short for me to enter fully into his way of thinking. My six years as an army doctor, working in special departments for brain injuries and injuries of the peripheral nervous system in Vienna, in neuropsychiatric wards of war hospitals and prisoner-of-war hospitals in Italy could not provide me with a clear theoretical orientation; rather, I obtained a certain training in improvisation and the conviction that nothing is impossible in human society. It would be dishonest to say that these experiences were always pleasant.

My work with Stransky did not influence my theoretical attitude. This was at that time more or less Freudian, whereas Stransky had for decades been a well-known enemy of psychoanalysis and a representative of an authoritarian psychotherapy and of classical psychiatry. Although his theories did not impress me very much, it was pleasant to work with a gentleman of the old tradition. Hans Hoff was very different, very dynamic, highly motivated to modernise Austrian neuropsychiatry, a very able manager for promoting the mental health movement. He also helped me greatly to obtain international experience, but there were sometimes severe scientific and personal tensions between us. What one could undoubtedly learn from him, nonetheless, was the value of his ruthless, dedicated efforts on behalf of general mental health.

At the same time a strong, indirect influence was exercised on me by August Aichhorn. When I commenced my psychoanalytical training he was too ill to take me into training analysis and he died shortly afterwards. Through the work of his pupils, for example Solms and Bolterauer, however, we came to learn something of his spirit and what we read and heard gave us a vivid picture of a person who was free to do what he felt necessary without any theoretical inhibitions.

In spite of my gratitude towards my three training-analysts – E. Schneider in Basel, A. Winterstein and Heilbrun in Vienna (all now, unfortunately, dead) – they did not influence me greatly in respect of my working orientation. The two psychoanalysts who impressed me considerably were E. H. Erikson and Anna Freud, though my contacts with both were limited. With some of the others I did not agree in every respect; to my surprise I found their perspective too narrow and the social viewpoint did not seem to exist for them.

Here I come to the social psychiatry, the second of my two legs, the first being psychotherapy, on which I have been standing for decades. The horrors of war and its political and racist persecution, and especially the experiences of nearly all my patients, made me aware of the role of politico-economic and social factors in health and illness and their impact on the selection of patients for therapy, the course of illness and the outcome of treatment. I therefore reacted strongly to the first reports from England and the United States on the new field of social psychiatry. I was the first to publish a book on this subject in German, with a series of studies in the field (Strotzka, 1958). The reaction to this volume was very poor, partly because it appeared too early for acceptance. My second book was the first systematic account of the discipline of social psychiatry in German (Strotzka, 1965) and became a considerable success, perhaps because it was published cheaply in pocket-book form.

A great influence on me was exercised by Anton Schimka, the former town planner of Vienna in the early 1950s, who was an ideal team partner, and by Leopold Rosenmayr, the first empirical sociologist to emerge in

Austria after the war. Fritz Redlich encouraged us strongly and also proved to be a very good friend.

In retrospect, however, I recognise that it was a group of institutions more than individuals which principally affected my attitudes and work. Of these I would enumerate the following.

(a) The World Federation of Mental Health and my associations with Otto Klineberg, Margaret Mead and the remarkable Sir Geoffrey Vickers. My unique experience as chairman of the Executive Board was immensely profitable.

(b) The National Institute of Mental Health, Bethesda, and my associations with Stanley Yolles, Bertram S. Brown and Morton Kramer. I received no research money from NIMH but a great deal of important and useful information.

(c) The Tavistock Institute, London, and my association with Henry Dicks, who introduced me to family therapy, John Bowlby, Michael Balint and David Malan.

(d) The Mental Health Division of the World Health Organisation in Geneva and Copenhagen, and my associations with Eduardo Krapf, Tsung Yi Lin and Donald Buckle; here I received wonderful working opportunities, especially the chance to participate in the work of the 'nuclear group' set up to reformulate the general classification of mental diseases.

(e) The Institute of Higher Studies (Ford Institute) in Vienna, gave me the necessary background to conduct two large epidemiological studies (Strotzka *et al.*, 1969), to write a book on mental health and well-baby clinics (Strotzka *et al.*, 1972), and to carry out studies on children in hospitals. Above all, I remember my debt to Dorli Simon in this sphere.

(f) H. E. Richter of the psychosomatic clinic at Giessen has been an influential friend and colleague and a pioneer in a psychoanalytically oriented social psychiatry and family therapy. Rarely does one find such harmony in parallel. Peter Fürstenau and some others have also figured prominently in these endeavours.

(g) Finally, in our own institute I would mention my good friend A. M. Becker, who works in the difficult field of psychoanalytical theory; Reiter, who studies values in psychotherapy and develops family therapy; and the many others who cooperated in our book on psychotherapy (Strotzka, ed. 1978) and have cooperated in the volume of case-studies and the study on institutions (1979 and 1980).

Here I would regard it as appropriate to comment on my religious, philosophical and humanistic outlook. With regard to religion the stiuation is straightforward: I am a non-believer but harbour no anti-religious sentiments. In philosophy Popper and Feigl (both of whom I have had the pleasure of meeting), Bertrand Russell and the young Topitsch, who wrote *Ursprung und Ende der Metaphysik*, have all been influential. The poetic sides of Nietzsche and Schopenhauer appeal greatly to me, and I have a certain liking not only for Montaigne but also for Machiavelli. My favourite books are Cervantes' *Don Quixote* and, with a sense of personal connection, Musil's *Man without Qualities*. I also like many important cartoonists from S. Steinberg to P. Flora. My musical interests are baroque, for example Bach, and contemporary composers such as Ligeti.

I think such interests have a certain importance and should not be omitted if one is bold enough to exhibit a self-portrait.

Current status of psychiatry

Public opinion of the present status of psychiatry is poor. To some extent it shares this position with general medicine, nuclear physics, biology and science as a whole. The wind is blowing against us. The 'anti-psychiatry' movement is not as strong as it was some years ago, but it can still be detected. Ivan Illich still recommends the abolition of all institutions, especially those associated with medicine and education; Thomas Szasz's views on psychiatry and mental illness and David Cooper's writings on the family are well-publicised; R. D. Laing claims that it is the non-schizophrenics who make up the mentally sick population. The younger generation buys and reads the books of all these people with great interest. The newspapers and magazines are filled with aggressive and bitter attacks against us psychiatrists.

Where does all this come from, and is it justified? Many antagonists of psychiatry are extremists with poor credentials for their judgements, whether they hold left-wing or right-wing opinions. However, there are other groups, including radical Christians and liberals of all persuasions, with a much better-informed background. Ecology is the only concept common to this group and, in general, the mass of their followers are deeply disappointed by the social situation in which they find themselves.

Some accusations against psychiatry are certainly justified. Many hospitals are still snake-pits of the worst kind. In many instances psychiatrists have apparently not been able to be consistently active and strong enough to force the authorities to change the situation to any extent. Too many have resigned and given up, escaping into biological research or phenomenological descriptions and have cared insufficiently for the deplorable conditions prevailing in their hospitals.

I myself, as a representative outpatient psychiatrist, felt relatively free from any responsibility for the situation within the psychiatric institutions, but this has not saved me from attack. I have been described as 'compromising' and reproached with being 'system immanent' or a 'progressive brakesman'. My answers to these accusations have been that I am sure that compromise is the only possible way of life in a democracy and that pluralism constitutes the only possibility of survival, but this response is not always taken seriously. Nonetheless, I can see no alternative to a rational approach, even from a non-committed position.

I understand that concepts of 'repressive tolerance' (H. Marcuse) and of 'structural violence' (Galtung) are regarded as signifying real progress in sociological theory. In consequence, psychiatry has to change; the effects of labelling and stigmatisation by psychiatric diagnosis have to be understood and taken into account. The general situation in psychiatry has to be changed by means of a combined effort drawing on money, energy and additional, better-qualified staff. On the other hand, to give up an interest in the basic issues of classification and nosology would lead to a reversion to the pre-scientific state of our discipline.

I am also sure that while psychiatric institutions are unavoidable for the general care of many patients, they have to be much smaller and better-run, preferably within the orbit of general hospitals. However, radical change – for example, towards part-time institutions or family-care – would sometimes impose too heavy a burden on families and society and make life for the patients even worse than it can be in a good open institution.

If, then, I try to summarise my impressions of the present status of psychiatry, the subject does not appear to be in good shape because psychiatrists themselves have not been able to improve the obviously bad conditions obtaining in their institutions. This knowledge has rendered them guilty in the eyes of their more extreme critics and there are few cogent arguments advanced by way of defence. Biological psychiatry has developed relatively quickly and well, but so far its impact on the well-being of psychiatric patients has not been impressive. Social psychiatry also made great strides but what appears to be satisfactory in theory is extremely slow and unsatisfying in practice. It is clearly not easy to change the mentality of either the personnel or the general public.

My personal concerns in this state of affairs are the following:

(a) I would be glad if I could contribute to a clarification of the nature of psychotherapy, to establish whether there are different indications for treatment and to distinguish between what must be considered as rational and scientific on the one hand and as pseudo-religious on the other.

(b) I try to remind our psychiatric colleagues that psychiatry means a concern not only for the major psychoses and psychiatric institutions but also for the so-called 'minor' psychiatric disorders which entail an enormous amount of suffering.

(c) I aim to improve the training standard of our health and social personnel in order to give them a better understanding and handling of psychosocial and psychosomatic problems and conflicts.

(d) The fourth and last point of concern is a little more complicated and needs more detailed consideration. I feel not only that the state of psychiatry and psychotherapy is alarming but that the general state of mankind gives rise for concern. It is hardly original to mention overpopulation, armaments and social justice in this context but, though it may seem banal to say so, it is astonishing that no strong and integrated action appears to have been taken. Medicine, and especially social medicine and psychiatry, should play an important part, together with political science, psychology and sociology, in developing strategies to counteract these dangers and to help the politician in his task. It seems obvious that the main barriers to action are psychological and that therefore these disciplines are relevant to the situation. In my opinion there is no longer any room for ivory towers in science. Curative and preventive action, teaching and research have to be *gesellschaftsrelevant* (socially relevant) in our field but – and this is extremely important – it must not be based on only *one* ideology but should be pluralistic. If politics can be conservative, liberal or socialist, so science should be basically open to *all* possible alternatives. In this sense my efforts can be compared with the activities of the Mitscherlichs and H. E. Richter in Germany and of P. Parin in Switzerland. If, as Clausewitz observed, *war* is the continuation of politics, the role has now fallen to *medicine*, as Virchow pointed out more than a century ago.

Future prospects of psychiatry

An attitude of resignation is probably the greatest sin in times of crisis. I shall not speculate further about world politics but confine myself to psychiatry and psychotherapy.

In psychotherapy the situation is particularly bad. There are grave doubts and uncertainties regarding definitions, indications, results, principles of action, organisation (for example within or outside universities), finance, legal issues, the concept of neurosis itself, professionalisation versus deprofessionalisation and, finally, the doubts concerning the need for psychotherapy at all.

Most disturbing of all is the large number of new methods being introduced as forms of psychotherapy. In my view all present psychotherapeutic concepts can be reduced to a few principles which have always been known to be effective in changing unwanted behaviour (see Table 1).

The need for psychotherapy should be decided, according to cultural customs, either by patient and therapist in *private* contracts or through the appropriate financing organisation (health service, insurance). The particular indication can be made on the basis of the personality, situation and illness of the patient, the abilities and situation of the therapist and, if it exists, the institution.

The development and training of a so-called 'basic psychotherapeutic attitude' on the part of the whole health and social personnel is most important. That means value-free acceptance, empathy, indirect counselling and sympathy. In this way the powerful but negative 'iatrogenic' influence of the current organically oriented medicine could be minimised. Self-help has to be encouraged, because most of the illnesses of civilisation can be best influenced by self-help groups, for example, alcoholism,

TABLE 1

1.	Training, learning, conditioning:	today known as behaviour modification
2.	Persuasion:	a permanent, but not always recognised principle
3.	Suggestion:	a permanent, well-recognised principle (autosuggestion + training = 'autogenous training')
4.	Counselling:	Rogerian therapy, social work
5.	Insight (making conscious):	all forms of depth psychology
6.	Group action:	group psychotherapy, group dynamics
7.	Systems-theory:	family therapy, communications therapy
8.	Abreaction, catharsis, ecstasis, meditation:	in some measure Gestalt therapy, psychodrama, encounter groups

obesity, lack of physical training and smoking. Psychotherapy should be practiced mainly by interdisciplinary and pluralistic teams, since only under such conditions can patient-centred goals and supervision be provided.

The possibility of the development of a new 'psychotherapy' profession based on an admixture of medical, psychological and social work training seems to me perhaps ideal for psychotherapy alone, but potentially dangerous because it could remove the concepts derived from psychotherapy from medicine altogether. This is a situation which has to be avoided in all circumstances.

For our present purpose it may be meaningless to discuss psychotherapy further, as the information needed to tackle the important administrative problems are related mainly to local circumstances and are of no general interest. I would prefer to pass on to a model of general psychiatric care. I feel that this could be of a didactic value because it lends itself to an overview of the connections between the population at risk with the different possibilities of treatment. This concept needs detailed discussion for its full development, but the outline shown in Fig. 1 indicates what I have in mind.

FIG. 1

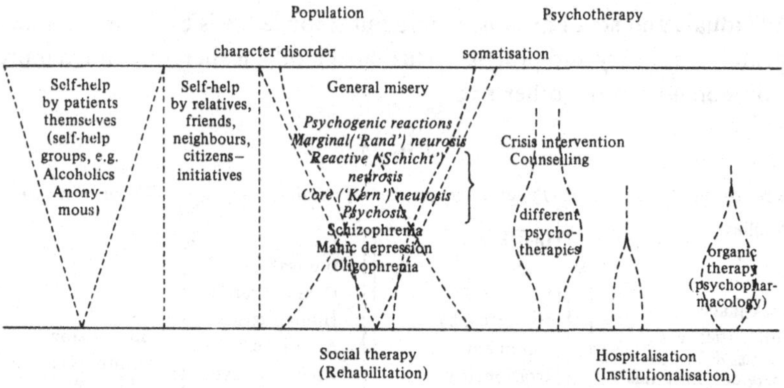

The model of psychiatric care has to be complemented by a model of prevention (Fig. 2). The concept of primary, secondary and tertiary sociogenesis had been worked out elsewhere. Primary sociogenesis signifies direct causation of disturbances by social conditions. Secondary sociogenesis means indirect causes, like poverty and oligophrenia, as an effect of bad nutrition, housing, lack of education and proper medical care. Tertiary sociogenesis refers to the influence of the environment on the course and outcome of all kinds of disturbances, depending on such factors as tolerance, acceptance, stigmatisation and segregation.

FIG. 2

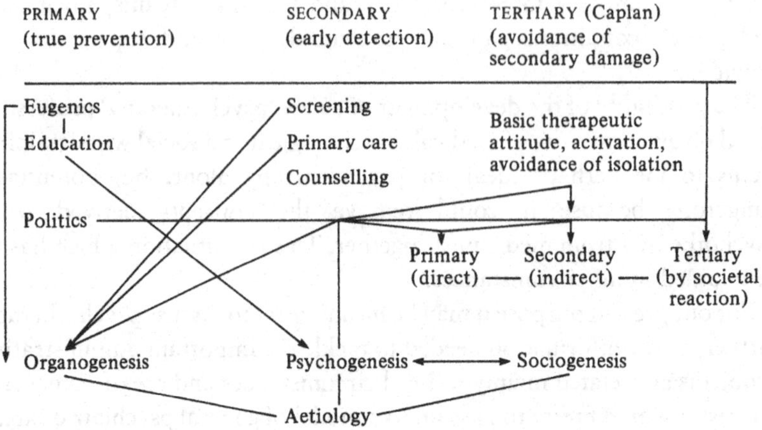

The central role of the political system, not only the health and social policy, becomes clear from this picture. However, the plan would not be complete without including the role of institutional care (Fig. 3). The problem posed by the institutions has become important as a result of the enormous increase of their role in modern society. Interaction and communication within them are sometimes more disturbed than between individuals and small groups, where our knowledge is based much more securely on theory and practice. This third model is therefore much more provisional than the other two.

FIG. 3

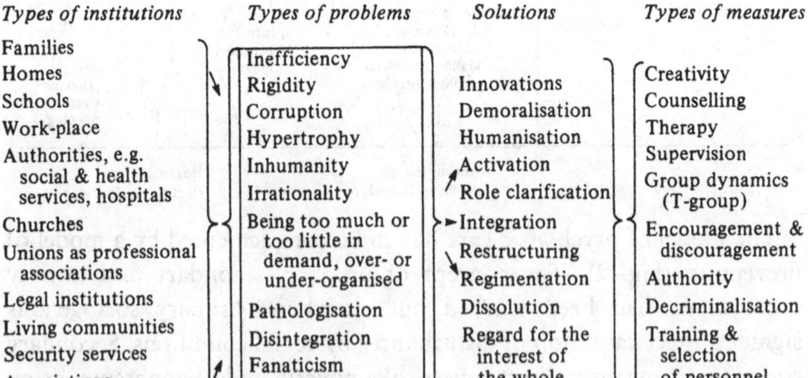

I would summarise my outlook on psychiatry as one of 'sceptical optimism'. I consider the improvement of the low status of psychiatry and psychotherapy today as one of the greatest unsolved problems in the western industrialised world. Basically, I feel that the problems are soluble. If this is so, the solutions may also be of benefit for larger world problems by leading to more humanity, rationality and understanding. The combination of a psychoanalytical attitude with social psychiatric experience may be a good basis on which to contribute a little in this direction.

Questions and answers

1. Why do you consider psychotherapy to be in a 'state of total chaos'?

I believe this to be the situation for several reasons.

(a) The arrival of so many new methods makes it almost hopeless to provide a comprehensive survey of the present situation. Most of these new methods and their underlying concepts are totally unscientific and remind me more of the activities and ideas of pseudo-religious sects than of rational treatment techniques. I believe that nearly all types of psychotherapy can be reduced to the few basic principles to which I have alluded. (p. 178).

(b) The lack of a clear definition imposes limits on the possibilities of education, indoctrination and all the other types of techniques designed to change behaviour. We have decided to formulate our definitions on the following axioms: (i) psychotherapy is a planned interaction between one or more patients and one or more therapists; (ii) it is used to treat behaviour disorders or states of suffering which are considered by a consensus as psycho- or socio-genic; (iii) the methods used should be teachable; (iv) the goals should be formulated; (v) the procedures should be based on a theory of normal and abnormal behaviour. The current theoretical orientations are mainly the learning theories, the psychoanalytical theories and the general systems theory. The various theories of philosophical anthropology at present seem to play a minor role.

(c) There are fundamental uncertainties about the organisation of psychotherapy. There is no general agreement as to who should treat whom and under which conditions. Nor is it clear whether a medical or other qualification is a prerequisite for a therapist; how the process of training should be professionalised; which clinical states call for treatment, for example there is a very common confusion between the neurosis in a narrower sense and the psychogenic reactions; what are the relative merits and demerits of single practice and team work; and how to clarify the roles of the traditional private scientific associations and the university departments.

(d) The uncertainties of financing make it difficult to decide whether psychotherapy should be covered by the state, by insurance companies or exclusively by private means. The sources of financial support for schemes also require elucidation.

(e) As a consequence of all these uncertainties in most countries the legal status of psychotherapy as a discipline and of its various schools is entirely open. After some experience with the new legal concepts in Germany and Austria for the regulation of these open questions I sometimes feel that a state of anarchy is preferable to the imposition of juridical regimentation.

All these factors constitute my justification for the word 'chaos'.

2. What is the present and future role of classical psychoanalysis?

The general impact of the unique work of Freud and most, or at least some, of his followers on all aspects of our culture is now widely acknowledged. Again and again new aspects of psychoanalytical theory emerge in surprising new contexts. Behaviour therapists and psychotherapists in the communist countries, for example Kabanow at the Bechterew Institute in Leningrad, are re-inventing transference and counter-transference. Whether the classical techniques should be adopted routinely, however, is more controversial. My personal impression with regard to the whole question – which is unavoidably not based on scientific grounds – is that psychoanalysis as a standard technique is still the best *training* method for most kinds of psychotherapy. Here the trainee learns introspection, empathy, insight into deeper emotions and, above all, patience in the face of regression and growth of his own and other personalities. For these reasons, it is also an important research method, but as a general method of treatment it is becoming very limited on two accounts: first, there are other very effective methods available and, secondly, the whole procedure is too expensive and consumes too much time and energy for general application. Professor Albert Stunkard, well-known for his outstanding work on the eating disorders, once said: 'If I want to understand an obese individual, I need psychoanalysis, but if I want to treat the obese, I need behaviour therapy and self-help groups.'

3. Will there be a place for psychotherapy in a scientific medicine?

This is the most difficult question of all and my answer must be still more tentative than those which I have already given.

What we call the 'basic psychotherapeutic attitude', which is very similar to the 'case-work attitude' in social work, has to be developed as strongly as possible as a counterweight against a more and more dehumanised technical medicine. This seems indisputable to me. We also have to fight against the very dangerous doctrine, nourished by the great power of the pharmaceutical industry, that medication is the answer to all forms of conflict and suffering. A 'psychosomatic' attitude has to be developed within all medical disciplines to counteract such tendencies.

At the same time there is a certain tendency for psychotherapy to develop out of medicine into psychology, social work and perhaps into a totally new profession. I am not unaware of some of the advantages which might arise from such a development, but in view of the overlapping areas of psychotherapeutic applications to the psychoses and the psychosomatic organic illnesses I would hope that psychotherapy will remain an integral part of medicine.

To keep psychotherapy within this framework a great deal has to be done to strengthen its scientific foundations. Much more empirical evaluation of outcome and process is needed than has been carried out hitherto. The work of such investigators as Lester Luborsky and Hans Strupp may be taken to indicate the way ahead. The increasing experience in the epidemiology of psychiatric illness, including the minor disorders, is very promising from the standpoint of method.

Select bibliography

Strotzka, H. & Navratil, L. (1954). Die Kind-Mutterrelation bei epileptischen Kindern. *Wiener Arch. PPN IV*.

Strotzka, H. (1955). Psychologische Probleme der Epilepsie. *Schweiz. Arch. Neur. Psych.*, 76.

Strotzka, H. (1956). Psychotherapie bei Phantomschmerzen. *Wiener Med. Wochenschrift*, **106**, 284–5.

Strotzka, H. (1956). Spannungen und Lösungsversuche in städtischer Umgebung. In *Wohnen in Wien*, ed. G. Krall, A. Schimka, L. Rosenmayr & H. Strotzka, pp. 94–109. Wien: Verlag für Jugend und Volk.

Strotzka, H. & Brodschöll, B. (1957). Statistische Untersuchungen zur Paranoiafrage. *Arch. Psych. und Z. Neur.*, **196**, 214–53.

Strotzka, H. (1958). *Sozialpsychiatrische Untersuchungen*. Wien: Springer Verlag.

Strotzka, H. & Förster, V. (1958). Sociometric investigation with Hungarian refugees as a basis for a mental health program. *Group Psychotherapy* XI, Dec. 1958.

Strotzka, H. (1965). *Einführung in die Sozialpsychiatrie.* Hamburg: Rde 214.

Strotzka, H. & Trappl, R. (1968). Kybernetische Modelle in der Psychiatrie. *Wiener Med. Wochenschrift*, **118**, 355–61.

Strotzka, H., Leitner, I., Czervenka-Wenkstetten, G., Graupe, S. & Simon , M. D. (1969). *Kleinburg, eine sozialpsychiatrische Feldstudie.* Wien: Österreichischer Bundesverlag.

Strotzka, H. (1969). *Psychotherapie und sociale Sicherheit.* Bern: Huber Verlag.

Strotzka, H. (1969). Psychotherapy for the working class. In *Social Psychiatry*, ed. F.C. Redlich. New York: Wilkins.

Strotzka, H. (1972). *Gesundheit für Millionen: Sozialpsychiatrie heute.* Wien & Hamburg: Paul Zsolnay Verlag.

Strotzka, H., Simon, M. D., Czermak, H. & Pernhaupt, G. (1972). *Psychotherapie und Mutterberatung.* Wien: Verlag für Jugend und Volk.

Strotzka, H. (1973). *Neurose, Charakter, soziale Umwelt. Beiträge zu einer speziellen Neurosenlehre.* (Geist und Psyche 2095.) München: Kindler.

Strotzka, H. (1973). Mental health aspects of camp clearance. (The activities of the mental health advisor to the UN High Commissioner for Refugees 1959/60.) *In Uprooting and After ...*, ed. S. Zwingmann & M. Pfister-Ammende, pp. 282–90. Berlin, Heidelberg & New York: Springer Verlag.

Strotzka, H. & Ligeti, V. (1973). Die Psychodynamik einer Gruppenregression. Psychoanalystische Beobachtungen bei jugendlichen Ungarnflüchtlingen. *Psyche*, 9, 870–85.

Strotzka, H. & Reiter, L. (1973). Some problems concerning the goals of psychotherapy. In *What is Psychotherapy?*, ed. J. Ruesch, San Francisco, California, A. H. Schmale, Rochester, New York, & Th. Spoerri, Bern. Proc. 9th Int. Congr. Psychotherapy, Oslo, 1973. Basel: S. Karger.

Strotzka, H. (1975). Hat die Psychotherapie in der Medizin der Zukunft noch einen Platz? *Wiener Med. Wochenschrift*, 125 Jg., 1–3.

Strotzka, H. (1975). Die gesellschaftliche Relevanz der Psychotherapie. In *Wissenschaft und Weltbild*, ed. W. Frühauf, pp. 497–508. Wien: Europaverlag.

Strotzka, H. (1976). Witz und Humor. In *Die Psychologie des 20. Jahrhunderts*, vol. II, ed. D. Eicke. Zürich: Kindler.

Strotzka, H. (ed.) (1978). *Psychotherapie* (2. Auflage), *Grundlagen, Verfahren, Indikationen.* München, Berlin, Wien: Urban & Schwarzenberg.

Strotzka, H. (1979). Die Rolle der Werte in der Entwicklung der Persönlichkeit. In *Werte Rechte Normen*, ed. Ansgar Paus, pp. 305–39. Styria Graz, Wien & Köln: Butzon & Bercker Kevelaer.

Strotzka, H. (1980). *Psychotherapeutische Feldstudien.* München: Urban und Schwarzenberg.

Strotzka, H. (1981). *Der Psychotherapeut im Spannungsfeld der Institutionen.* München: Urban und Schwarzenberg.

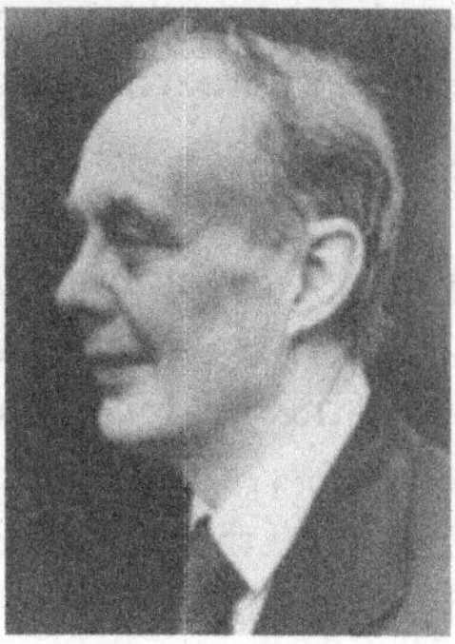

12 · DAVID WATT

Personal background and professional experience

My medical undergraduate training started in 1937 at Glasgow University. The Scottish system allowed students to choose their teachers from a number of city and outlying hospitals associated with the university. I intended to go into general practice and gave special attention to obstetrics, paediatrics and dermatology. For one summer vacation I worked in a subnormality hospital. The experience was a considerable shock. Undergraduate training was directed towards acute hospital-based illness, comprehensible in biological terms, which did not encompass severe, permanent incapacity or provide a base for a constructive orientation towards these grotesque variants of human form and function. I hardly encountered psychiatry as a student, except in the writings of Morton Prince, Freud and Bernard Hart.

After 18 months of hospital medicine and obstetrics, I worked in general practice, where the frequency of psychiatric illness was quickly forced on my attention. The nearest psychiatric hospital was 30 miles away; there were no outpatient clinics. The added exigencies of war-time made psychiatric consultation impossible and with my lack of practical experience textbook consultation was unenlightening. I therefore took a six-month job at the Royal Mental Hospital in Glasgow. The regime of hospitals in Britain then was moulded by the statutory requirements of the Lunacy Act and 'voluntary' patients were the minority. Nevertheless, the psychobiological principles of Adolf Meyer, largely mediated through the standard British textbook of the period (Henderson & Gillespie), formed the framework for a medical approach which supported systematic observation of symptoms, related them to life history and encouraged orderly case-reporting.

My next appointment was in a newly built hospital 30 miles outside London but serving a catchment area in West London, which extended from the northern outskirts to the Thames. The clinical work of junior staff was based on acute admissions rather than chronic cases, a departure from the widely accepted practice of the period. Electroconvulsive therapy had become an established treatment for inpatient depressive illness but, because of its physical rigours, many common somatic disorders were a bar to treatment. I was able to explore and reassess these drawbacks when the treatment was modified by application of the newly discovered muscle relaxants and this formed the basis for a doctorate thesis and first publication (Watt & Shepherd, 1949).

After a short course in neurology, I was attracted by the training opportunities at the Maudsley Hospital during the early period of its post-war expansion and spent three years there. The backbone of clinical training was the systematic, intensive case-work instituted by Aubrey Lewis who, as a teacher, was such a brilliant exponent of the method. This was supplemented by a period of child psychiatry and of psychotherapy in both inpatient and outpatient settings.

On leaving the Maudsley in 1952 I became a consultant at St John's Hospital, Aylesbury, where I now work. My career as a psychiatrist has therefore been spent almost wholly in mental hospitals during a period which overlaps the introduction of the National Health Service.

A striking improvement in psychiatric services took place in the decade following the inception of the National Health Service. This was typified by the changes in St John's Hospital. Opened in 1853, it was conceived in the light of the humane ideas of the period, a sound and modern building (Pevsner, 1960) placed at the centre of Buckinghamshire in a beautiful situation looking southwards to the Chiltern Hills. The growth of fundamental knowledge on which medicine and surgery advanced so rapidly from the end of last century was not matched by comparably spectacular results in psychiatry and the disappointment generated may have contributed to its neglect during the first third of this century. The arousal of St John's Hospital from this torpid period in the mid-1930s by the Medical Superintendent, Dr I. Skottowe, a vigorous and forward-looking administrator, with effects that anticipated many of the national changes of the post-war period, has been documented in a detailed study of the changes in the St John's population over this time (Shepherd, 1957). Although larger plans were frustrated by the war, a foundation had been laid which provided a jumping off point for post-war development. During the decade from 1952, with Dr S. L. Last as Medical Superintendent, the neglect of 40 years and two wars was repaired in an ambitious scheme of improving and transforming the main buildings; the opening of a purpose-built admission unit, a unit in a local general hospital and a day hospital; the creation or enlargement of social work, psychology and occupational therapy services as well as an increasing and reorganisation of the nursing and medical staff.

The first of the modern tranquilising drugs, reserpine, introduced to Western countries in 1953 was in fact a plant extract with a calming effect used in Indian ayurvedic medicine for centuries. In the earliest controlled clinical trial we found that it had limited value in schizophrenia (Watt & Shepherd, 1956; Watt, 1956) but was effective both in controlling and shortening attacks of mania (Watt, 1958). Animal experiments showed striking effects in learning and perception (Weiskrantz & Wilson, 1955; Weiskrantz, 1957) and it was a logical step to explore these psychological properties in human subjects as a possible explanation of its therapeutic action (Watt & Crookes, 1961; Watt, Allport & Crookes, 1964; Watt, Crookes & McDonald, 1966). Having worked as a consultant for 10 years, I succeeded Dr Last as Medical Director in 1962.

While the improvement in psychiatric services in the first decade of the National Health Service can be partly attributed to the general recovery from post-war conditions, I nevertheless believe that, while taking into account inherent drawbacks, the Health Service gives the best framework for the practice and progress of psychiatry. Private practice fosters an item-of-service individualistic approach from the doctor, whereas psychiatry requires continuity and team-work. Where private practice is predominant, research and training, the keys to the development of psychiatry, are almost inevitably neglected.

In view of the progress made in patient care at St John's, it seemed to me that the aims of establishing research and training as accepted mental hospital responsibilities and activities should be given priority. An opportunity to pursue the first of these aims rapidly presented itself. The new admission wing opened in 1960 contained a purpose-built unit for insulin coma therapy of schizophrenia. This procedure, originally introduced for serious drug addiction by Sakel in 1934 and then becoming a specific treatment for schizophrenia, had been virtually abandoned by 1960 following the discovery of the phenothiazine drugs and the advent of psychopharmacology. The new unit was therefore conveniently converted into a biochemistry laboratory for psychopharmacological research and has been continuously used for the investigation of schizophrenia and depressive illness. Research as part of their activities has always been an option open to clinical consultants within the Health Service. In a specialty lacking a foundation in basic sciences but as important as psychiatry, research becomes a pressing responsibility. In practice, however, service needs are so clamant that it seldom receives its share. With this in mind, the consultant vacancy created by my promotion was advertised with time allocated to research and written into the appointee's contract. Difficult to preserve as is this small investment of time, it has catalysed continuous research activity at a point where the need is most obvious and the material most abundant (for example Crammer & Scott, 1966; Bond & Cundall, 1977).

Until 1960 the large majority of psychiatrists in Britain were trained in mental hospitals 'on the job' by individual clinical supervision from consultants, of whom only a small number undertook this task in a systematic way. To make up for the deficiency I initiated short courses open to medical staff of all psychiatric hospitals in the local region as a preliminary step in systematic instruction, supplementing hospital teaching and allowing a comparison of standards between hospitals by the trainees themselves. A committee of representatives from each hospital, the prototype for clinical tutors in psychiatry, organised these and other postgraduate training activities. In 1972 I became the Chairman of the newly formed Clinical Tutors' Sub-Committee of the Royal Medico-Psychological Association, which fostered a similar effort on a national scale. During the period of adumbration of the Royal College of Psychiatrists, the Clinical Tutors' Committee was able to bring the aspirations of trainees to bear on College planning, particularly in modifying the domination of the training period by the examination for membership of the College and by promoting continuous clinical training through the inspection and accreditation of individual hospitals, thus securing general adoption of at least minimal agreed standards.

Current status of psychiatry

British mental hospitals emerged from the last war with no living tradition of humane care to replace that which had inspired their building. Further, they were bound by outdated legal constraints which choked all impulses towards improvement. The advent of the National Health Service in 1949, aspiring to provide medical care to whomever needed it, furnished the stimulus and opportunity for change. An accidental benefit was the abolition of the legal distinction between private and 'rate-aided' patients which had subjected the latter class to the humiliation of discharge by a lay management committee. The uniform grading of medical staff throughout the NHS, which removed the financial disincentive for recruitment into mental hospitals, was a more calculated asset. The establishment of Regional Hospital Boards allowed a planned improvement of mental hospitals and an expansion of services. Following a Royal Commission report, which remains the most comprehensive review of mental illness policy this century, a more flexible and practical legal framework was provided in the Mental Health Act of 1959. During the early 1960s the fruits of these changes appeared as a comprehensive system of varied forms of care centred upon the psychiatric hospital, from which began to emerge a coherent system of training for doctors, nurses and social workers, together with a working method of bringing their complementary skills to bear on the problems of care, assessment, treatment, rehabilitation and support of the heterogeneous groups of ill and maladjusted people for whom they assumed responsibility.

Albeit unevenly, psychiatric hospitals achieved a remarkable transformation and adaptation of their services to meet the new demands. Unfortunately this progress did not continue, as the distressing sequence of official inquiries into mental hospitals during the last decade harshly attests. In seeking the causes of this decline we are assisted by the Department of Health's appraisal *Better Services for the Mentally Ill* (HMSO, 1975) which has conveniently identified many of the landmarks. The first of these was the publication (Tooth & Brooke, 1961) of a prediction that 'none of the patients then in hospital would still be there in 15 years or so', with the consequent assumption that the short-term treatment of acute illness would be the only task of the psychiatric service. This forecast, obtained by a linear projection of the observation that between 1954 and 1960 occupied beds in mental hospitals had dropped from 3.4 to 3.1 per 1,000 of the population, was immediately criticised on two grounds. The first, a criticism of the statistical method, was based on the argument that a linear projection was not appropriate (Norton, 1961; Kingston, 1963); and the second was founded on the argument that there were in any case good reasons for believing that the decline in mental hospitals numbers would not continue (Gore & Jones, 1961; Brooke, 1962; Rollin, 1963; Watt, 1963a, 1963b, 1967a, 1967b).

The driving force behind belief in a continued decline of the long-stay population of mental hospitals with termination of recruitment to its numbers, however, was the conviction that the use of 'modern' drugs would effect the miracle. A study of St John's Hospital's statistics, both in the year preceding and those following the introduction of tranquilisers (Shepherd, Goodman, & Watt, 1961), has an important bearing on this issue. The drugs in question came into general use around 1955. Between 1954 and 1957, the number of hospital admissions, discharges and the proportion of readmissions rose markedly, mainly in respect of neurosis and affective disorders. Among schizophrenics, however, where the greatest effect of tranquilising drugs might have been anticipated, there was no change in the numbers admitted, discharged or resident. There was a slight rise in the total resident population and no change in the proportion of long-stay patients. The increase in admissions, discharges and the proportion of readmissions was seen to be the continuation of a trend dating from the mid-1940s resulting from hospital policy encouraging early discharge and extramural care.

This aspect of declining hospital numbers was underlined by the results of several studies: an increased discharge rate following the introduction of psychotropic drugs was shown to occur not only among the treated but also among untreated cases (Linn, 1959); and psychotropic drugs have a more limited effect on discharge rates where a favourable environment and active rehabilitation programmes have already been created (Rathod, 1958). Shepherd's earlier study (1957) of St John's Hospital showed in the pre-drug era the dramatic effect of an enlightened policy in shortening hospital stay and increasing the discharge rate, and a later study, also at St John's Hospital, indicated the powerful influence of preserved family bonds, particularly marriage and other social determinants, on the prospects of discharge from prolonged hospital stay (Watt & Buglass, 1966). In the light of these factors, the decline in hospital resident numbers would obviously precede an inevitable flattening out as the slack is taken up.

Although events have proved the validity of these criticisms, the original prediction has nevertheless remained the foundation of government policy, according to which acute psychiatric illness calls for provision only in general hospital units, with 'community care' support. The Secretary of State in 1975, for instance, in her foreword to *Better Services for the Mentally Ill* (1975), stated:

> Specialist care is still mainly based in large geographically isolated mental hospitals.... There have, of course, been some improvements

> and changes. . . . But these improvements are not getting to the core of the problem. What we have to do is to get to grips with shifting the emphasis to community care. Social service facilities – hostels, day centres, group homes – have to be built up . . . . Staff to run them have to be recruited and trained . . . . Psychiatric services have to be developed locally, in general and community hospitals and in health centres.

Unfortunately, several jarring notes disturb the harmony of this broad scheme. The report goes on to say:

> The term 'open door hospital' has like 'community care' become with time something of a catch phrase . . . . What is required is a service which is flexible and capable of dealing at local level, whenever possible, with the difficult behaviour and violence which may occur from time to time during treatment of particular patients . . . . We need to revive the interest in meeting the needs of long-stay patients in a way which is challenging and satisfying for both staff and patients, and which integrates such care with that of the shorter-stay patients instead of regarding it almost as a separate and often second-tier service . . . .

The question that these problems pose is whether, as the document assumed, 'they are at the margin and that the basic concept remains valid'. At the margin or at the centre, the effect on mental hospitals of these afterthoughts on policy is considerable; long-stay and psychogeriatric patients, and those with 'difficult behaviour and violence which may occur from time to time', all remain their responsibility.

In 1973 the reorganisation of the administration of the Health Service took place, its prime object was to coordinate hospital, general practitioner and local authority health services. The legacy of this upheaval for mental hospitals is an unwieldy form of administration unsuited to their needs, based as it is on the conception of a comprehensive district general hospital. Most mental hospitals serve several districts, each having an administration which focuses its main effort on its district hospital. Medical, nursing and other essential services are therefore administered remotely from the mental hospital and rarely by officers having experience of the care of psychiatric patients and hospitals. Within hospitals erosion of medical leadership has left a vacuum in initiative and responsibility. Their destructive results have been lucidly identified by a doctor and lawyer who, having conducted two mental hospital official enquiries, have had a unique opportunity to give an informed outsider's view (Inskip & Edwards, 1979). They observe that 'the total care of a patient embraces diagnosis, physical treatments, accommodation, furnishing, clothing, feeding, occupation, and much else' but that it is unclear for which of these 'the medical officer is solely responsible, in the sense that he alone has the knowledge to arrive at an informed decision'. They attribute this to the action of the Department of Health and Social Security in 'sweeping away the old system of physician superintendent, which with all its faults had at least a clearly understood chain of command', and failing to replace it with a clearly identified source of authority and responsibility.

Turning to the movement of patient populations in psychiatric hospitals and units, the most recent national assessment (DHSS, 1978) gives a surprising picture of the proportion of the load taken by psychiatric hospitals after 15 years of rundown. In the decade from 1964 admissions to general hospital units have more than doubled (23,000 to 48,000) but in the same period admissions to mental hospitals have altered by less than 5 per cent (128,000 to 121,000). Seventy per cent of all psychiatric admissions still go to mental hospitals which, it is clear, deal with the bulk of serious psychiatric illness.

What has been the effect on mental hospitals of modern treatments? Therapeutic innovations since the end of the war have been the establishment of ECT and the introduction of antidepressive drugs and major and minor tranquillisers. Psychologists have introduced treatments dependent on learning theory and there has been a substantial increase in our knowledge of social causes bearing on major psychiatric illness. Mental hospitals have become more open and extramural services have increased. From the clinical viewpoint considerable improvement appears to have resulted, insofar as major illnesses are less painful to bear and easier to manage; the quality of life of psychiatric patients has become better. National figures (DHSS, 1978) for the decade up to 1975, however, give little evidence of an impact on psychiatric inpatient numbers. Admissions have risen to fill the greater accommodation available and readmissions have increased. A greater proportion of patients spend less than one month in hospital, but there is no decrease in the proportion who stay longer than one year.

It is clear that present therapy is palliative and knowledge of the aetiology of major psychiatric illness is needed to provide the basis for radical curative and preventive measures. In the meantime the evaluation of each innovation in treatment by methods which give decisive answers is the only way of testing for firm ground. Nowhere is this more true than in the changes which have been adopted in the care and treatment of schizophrenia. The introduction in the mid-1960s of long-acting drugs in slow-release preparations given by injection has been accompanied by a widely adopted system of oversight of discharged patients by experienced psychiatric nurses who administer the injections. St John's Hospital, situated as it is at the centre of a well-demarcated, stable population, which it serves by schizophrenic follow-up clinics in the surrounding local general hospitals, is particularly well-placed for the evaluation of the separate elements of this change. The introduction of an oral long-acting preparation (pimozide) as a treatment in schizophrenia provided the opportunity for this to be done. It was shown that not only was oral administration as effective clinically as parenteral medication (Falloon, Watt & Shepherd, 1978*a*) but, surprisingly, in the evaluation of patients' social functioning it proved superior (Falloon, Watt & Shepherd, 1978*b*), possibly through greater flexibility in the adjustment of the dose to reduce socially handicapping side-effects.

Future prospects of psychiatry

It appears from recent trends that mental hospitals will be responsible for the care and treatment of the bulk of serious mental illness for the calculable future and that their morale and standard of service have declined. I believe two conditions must be met to arrest the decline and enhance the contribution of mental hospitals. The first is that the contradictions of the present national policy must be removed and replaced by a consistent plan; the second is that the mental hospitals must have more effective individual administration and leadership. Mental hospitals are pressed to move in several directions at once. They must be therapeutically active, welcoming, reassuring, scrupulous in respecting individual freedom, 'open' and moving towards 'community care', at the same time as they are urged not to be reluctant to accept patients with difficult behaviour problems and to be prepared to develop a service which is 'flexible and capable of dealing at local level, wherever possible, with the difficult behaviour and violence which may occur from time to time' (HMSO, 1975). In addition, mental hospitals house practically all seriously demented patients whose frailty, nursing dependence, numbers and outcome make their needs conflict severely with those of other patient groups. How are such contortionist feats of orientation, allocation of staff and disposition of buildings to be performed? The most basic policy contradiction, however, is the thesis of the *Hospital Plan for England and*

Wales (HMSO, 1962) on which present policy is founded. *Better Services for the Mentally Ill* (the 1975 statement of DHSS policy) refers to the 1961 projection of numbers in mental hospitals as if it had largely been fulfilled, except for a little raggedness at the edges, and were still a valid basis for present planning (para. 2, 15, p. 16). It says, for instance, 'what has actually happened is that a substantial number of patients who were in hospital in 1954, the data basis used for the 1961 projections, are still there. In 1971 some 30,000 of the original 110,000 __patients resident for more than 2 years_ were still in hospital'. This statement is so irrelevant as to be misleading in the context of this argument: there were 67,000 psychiatric inpatients resident for more than two years in England alone in 1971 (DHSS, 1978).

A conspicuous deficiency in the administration of psychiatric hospitals is the lack of psychiatric experience in Health Service administrative staff – administrators, community physicians, nursing and personnel officers – at district, area and regional levels. This is also true of the social services (Jones, 1979). The system of advisors or advisory committees, which is the improvised method of dealing with this lack, is inadequate because it does not allow the continuous review of business which would prompt initiative or scrutiny of planning in the knowledge of psychiatric practice and requirements.

The foremost medical task for psychiatry in the future is the application of known and accepted treatments to mental illness, with rehabilitation and care an important second priority. At present these procedures are empirical; knowledge and skill in their application are derived from experience and judgement and it is clear that judgements vary considerably. Hence the importance that psychiatrists, in both the period of training and of responsibility, should constantly be exposed to varying responsible opinions and be called on to justify their own viewpoints and decisions in day-to-day practice, at academic meetings and during the interchanges organised by professional bodies. Psychiatric practice and opinion need exposure to the scrutiny, co-operation and alliance of other disciplines, both biological and social. While academic centres are the main generators of such ferment, its importance within mental hospitals, where the majority of psychiatrists are trained, is equally obvious.

Progress towards a rational basis for psychiatry is slow, dependent as it is on the disproportion between research done and the size of the problem. We have, for example, no plausible explanation of the therapeutic action of ECT, an effective treatment in widespread use for 40 years; anorexia nervosa, recognised for 50 years, has no accepted aetiology or reliable treatment. Relatively few psychiatrists emerge with the ability and will to lay claim on the time and resources which research requires. This is perhaps attributable to the lack of stimulation and example in mental hospitals where little research is done but most psychiatrists are trained.

Progress in psychiatry will depend in large measure on its ability to attract able doctors. It is at present noticeably lacking in appeal to newly qualified graduates in several countries, including the United Kingdom, where many hospitals are dependent for their junior medical staff on Commonwealth doctors or on clinical assistants and trainees from general practice. Married women seeking part-time training in a fixed locality have provided a vitalising transfusion to many hospitals. Their training is often submerged by service needs, however, and the attainment of a satisfying career subsequently seems exceptional and fortuitous.

No less important for the well-being of the psychiatric hospital is the presence of other staff services to patients. Nurses are most directly influential in the administration of treatment, care and rehabilitation. Of the many conditions necessary for maintaining quality and numbers, a vigorous and independent training school is indispensable. In present conditions, however, it is hampered and devitalised by the 'line management' concept whereby it is a sub-section of the 'district' training school, administered remotely from its parent hospital. Psychiatric social workers form the link in effecting the continuation of care from hospital to community. To contribute effectively they must be able to comment on and draw from assessment and treatment planning of all patients from the time of first contact with the hospital. The present administrative structure does little to nourish these conditions, and few hospitals in the post-war period have been able to maintain this vital service continuously. Although occupational therapy in relation to psychiatry has not been informed by such a clear philosophy as in other specialties, for example orthopaedics, the value of a flexible and imaginatively run service undoubtedly helps to prevent secondary impairment, to promote training and educational experience for psychiatric patients and to maintain the satisfaction of social function despite disability.

It is apparent that both psychiatric hospitals and psychiatric units in general hospitals can treat and care for serious mental disorder, each possessing advantages and drawbacks according to local situation and circumstances. It is equally clear that the aim to replace all psychiatric hospitals with such units is a will o' the wisp venture which misdirects and dissipates the energy and resources which psychiatry so urgently needs.

David Watt

Questions and answers

1. In view of the argument you advance concerning the continued importance of the mental hospital, what specific measures would you recommend to improve working conditions in these institutions?

Measures to improve working conditions in mental hospitals must start with the delineation of a consistent policy as the foundation for reasonable administration, bearing in mind the considerable areas for which there is no consensus on purpose and practice. There are, nevertheless, measures which would improve mental hospitals in the performance of the functions which they now undertake. These institutions need an administration linked to but distinct from that of other hospitals. At every level of administration (district, area and region) the officers should have substantial working experience of psychiatric and subnormality hospitals (i.e. as much experience as they have of general hospitals), including the areas of medical and general administration, nursing, personnel, works, finance, pharmacy and catering, as long as 'line management' persists as the doctrine of hospital administration.

All psychiatric hospitals (or services) should have a medical administrator: the heir to but not in the mould of the medical superintendent. He should be a working clinician for at least half his time, without clinical jurisdiction over his consultant colleagues. He should initiate the formulation of medical policy, promulgate it and co-ordinate it with nursing, social work and other areas of hospital function. He should initiate consultation and action as need arises and act as spokesman and representative of his medical colleagues, particularly in relation to lay administration.

Reducing the humiliation most people feel at being admitted to mental hospitals is an important item in improving institutional public relations. This is partly due to the nature of serious psychiatric illnesses, which often affect judgement and capacity for appropriate social behaviour and from which unaffected people feel they are immune. More than this, however, people encounter in psychiatric hospitals a demoralising departure from domestic standards to which they are accustomed, one which is offensive to them in matters of cleanliness, privacy, diet, amenity and comfort, all resulting from the scanty funds and services which psychiatric hospitals suffer and representing a legacy of the dependence on patients for domestic work, now rightly condemned and withdrawn but without organised replacement. For this reason psychiatric hospitals should consistently receive a fixed proportion of the available budget, related primarily to the size of their catchment area population and the nature of the services they render, for example psychogeriatrics, long stay and community support.

A deplorable feature of clinical practice in mental hospitals is the lack of standardisation in collecting and recording information. This is a severe hindrance to clinical, research and administrative practice. The remedial measures which could be applied are neglected: I would suggest the following three initially:

(a) the use throughout mental hospitals of the World Health Organisation glossary of mental disorders (1978);
(b) the use of a standard format for taking clinical histories and recording case-notes;
(c) the creation of a clinical standardisation committee by the Royal College of Psychiatrists to investigate and advise on these matters.

2. How do you view the social and community psychiatry movement which has been so widely publicised in recent years?

The phrase 'social and community psychiatry movement' covers three areas: (a) the social causes of psychiatric illness; (b) the phenomena of group illness or disturbance; and (c) the social and community treatment of psychiatric illness. Each has a long history within psychiatry, but often a revival of interest in a particular aspect emerges with a new name. During the last decade attention directed to 'life events', for instance, can be seen as an attempt to render more precise the long-standing idea of 'reactive illness'. The concept of most relevance to psychiatric hospitals which has been recently publicised, however, is the social and community treatment of psychiatric illness.

The hard-won recognition in the 1920s of psychiatric social work as a speciality requiring its own training and experience attests the recognition and importance attached to social investigation and support in psychiatry. This preceded their recognition in other medical specialities, even at a time when psychiatry was almost wholly hospital-based. A major social effect of hospitalisation for mental illness then was the loss to family life of the wage-earner or parent and the impairment of life prospects for the child. Community psychiatry, by substituting treatment and support at home, attempts to preserve the bonds and to resolve tensions in family life which are seen as playing a major part in the cause or precipitation of the psychiatric illness. The movement has received strong official impetus as a more economical way of dealing with psychiatric illness. Whatever advantage this arrangement may have, however, it transfers the onus of living with and supporting patients to relatives, with consequent strain or impoverishment of family resources and relationships. Currently accepted but invalidated theories of the social causes of schizophrenia (Leff, 1978) fasten responsibility for the illness on spouses, parents or children, placing on them an additional burden of blame and guilt.

A more moderate view sees community psychiatry as extending treatment with a variety of supplements to a hospital-based service: patient clubs, sheltered workshops, day-hospitals, halfway houses, hostels, group homes. The most constant observation on these facilities in Britain is that their provision is inadequate. It seems likely that they cater largely for psychiatric disorders which differ from those customarily admitted for inpatient care, as it is clear that their introduction has not affected inpatient admissions. They also operate as a resource additional to inpatient treatment, particularly in output of rehabilitation and resettlement. In the last decade St John's Hospital has instituted several group homes, each housing up to six self-supporting patients, who would otherwise be permanently resident; they are prepared for this transfer by a period in a resettlement flat in the hospital. An important feature of this arrangement, however, is the deployment of psychiatrically skilled personnel, of whom social workers are the most representative, and it is the revival of these activities closely integrated with those of psychiatrists and nurses, which seems to me the indispensable condition for a useful role for the social and community psychiatry movement.

3. What forms of research can be most profitably pursued in mental hospitals at the present time?

The obvious potential of mental hospitals in psychiatric research is an abundance of clinical material, particularly the psychoses. The most notable contributions to our contemporary understanding of this group of illnesses, from Kraepelin and Bleuler to *Schizophrenia and Social Care* (Brown *et al.*, 1966), have come from work in mental hospitals and this remains the area of mental hospital research from which the greatest yield may be anticipated. Since the psychoses have become an important field of pharmaceutical interest the evaluation of treatment by clinical trials has become a pressing preoccupation in psychiatry. The Medical Research Council (MRC) trial of the treatment of depressive illness (1965) could have produced its results in no other way than as a co-operative venture involving 60 mental hospitals, and it remains the major controlled clinical trial of ECT in depressive illness, as well as a landmark in establishing the efficacy of the two groups of anti-depressive drugs employed. Multicentre trials consume such large resources in organisation and co-ordination that projects within single hospitals are preferable where they are appropriate, as in the trial of prostaglandin suppression in schizophrenia completed at St John's Hospital (Falloon *et al.*, 1978). Specialist facilities are seldom situated in mental hospitals but in Britain they have been very productive, as with the MRC Unit in Graylingwell Hospital, the Kennedy–Galton genetics unit in Harperbury Hospital and the neuropathology departments in Runwell and the Fountain hospitals. The biochemistry laboratory established in St John's Hospital has facilitated the substantial use of clinical material for combined clinical and biochemical investigations (for example, Watt, Crammer & Elkes, 1972; Crammer & Scott 1966; Bond & Cundall, 1977).

It is notable that many research bodies concerned with psychiatry give a disproportionately small share of their funds to clinical research compared with purely laboratory and animal work; this must be attributed in part to the negligible research expertise and resources available in mental hospitals. Research bodies should, in my opinion, do more specifically to fertilise and nourish research in mental hospitals. A modest sustained provision of expertise in neurochemistry, genetics, epidemiology, statistics, neurophysiology, neurohistology or endocrinology with specialised research wards (for example, metabolic) would transform this situation. Clinical psychology units in psychiatric hospitals were a prolific source and sustenance of clinical research until in recent times psychologists found a new role as therapists rather than as investigators. Academic psychiatric units have provided stimulation and guidance for research but their own resources are meagre and they frequently limit their interest to the plundering of research material or supplementary staff from mental hospitals. The Scandinavian model, where academic departments are based in psychiatric hospitals, deserves a trial elsewhere.

Neglect of the evaluation of services has a noticeable effect on psychiatric practice. Each innovation becomes a panacea, so that we lurch from 'open hospital' to 'secure unit', or from 'early admission' to 'crisis intervention', with little learned from each change in fashion and occasionally, as in the move to units in district general hospitals, a vast dissipation of resources. The comparison of three different types of mental hospital regime carried out by Brown and his colleagues (1966) indicates how, as well as evaluating these different approaches, valuable clinical knowledge can also be gained. The flexibility shown by mental hospital staff, particularly nurses, in adapting themselves to provide varying modes of care presents the opportunity for the weighing value against the cost of each.

References

Bond, P. A. & Cundall, R. L. (1977). Properties of monoamine oxidase (MAO) in human blood platelets, plasma, lymphocytes and granulocytes. *Clinica Chimica Acta*, 80, 317–26.

Brooke, E. (1962). Factors affecting the demand for psychiatric beds. *Lancet*, ii, 1211–13.

Brown, G. W., Bone, M., Dalison, B. & Wing, J. K. (1966). Schizophrenia and Social Care. London: Oxford University Press.

Crammer, J. L. & Scott, B. (1966). The excretion of desmethylimipramine and its metabolites in depressive patients. Proceedings of IV World Congress of Psychiatry. *Excerpta Medica International Congress Series No. 150*, 1942–44.

Department of Health and Social Security (1978). In-patient statistics from the mental health enquiry for England, 1975. HMSO.

Falloon, I., Watt, D. C., Lubbe, K., Macdonald, A. & Shepherd, M. (1978). N-acetyl-p-amino-phenol (paracetamol aceteminophen) in the treatment of schizophrenia. *Psychological Medicine*, 8, 495–9.

Fallon, I., Watt, D. C. & Shepherd, M. (1978*a*). A comparative controlled trial of pimozide and fluphenazine decanoate in the continuation therapy of schizophrenia. *Psychological Medicine*, 8, 59–70.

Falloon, I., Watt, D. C. & Shepherd, M. (1978*b*). The social outcome of long-term continuation therapy in schizophrenia: pimozide vs. fluphenazine. *Psychological Medicine*, 8, 265–74.

Gore, C. P. & Jones, K. (1961). Survey of a long-stay mental hospital population. *Lancet*, ii, 544–6.

HMSO (1962). *Hospital Plan for England and Wales*.

HMSO (1975). *Better Services for the Mentally Ill*.

Inskip, J. H. & Edwards, J. G. (1979). Mental hospital enquiries. *Lancet*, i, 658–60.

Jones, K. (1979). Integration or disintegration in the mental health services. *Journal of the Royal Society of Medicine*, 72, 640–8.

Kingston, F. E. (1963). The demand for psychiatric beds. (Letter.) *Lancet*, i, 107–8.

Leff, J. (1978). Social and psychological causes of the acute attack. In *Schizophrenia: Towards a New Synthesis*, ed. J. K. Wing. London: Academic Press.

Linn, E. L. (1959). Drug therapy, milieu change, and release from a mental hospital. *Archives of Neurology and Psychiatry*, 81, 785–94.

Medical Research Council (1965). Clinical trial of the treatment of depressive illness. *British Medical Journal*, i, 881–6.

Norton, A. (1961). The demand for psychiatric beds. (Letter.) *Lancet*, i, 884.

Pevsner, N. (1960). *The Buildings of England — Buckinghamshire*. London: Penguin Books.

Rathod, N. H. (1958). Tranquilisers and patient's environment. *Lancet*, i, 611–13.

Rollin, H. R. (1963). The demand for psychiatric beds. (Letter.) *Lancet*, i, 386.

Shepherd, M. (1957). *A Study of the Major Psychoses in an English County*. London: Chapman & Hall.

Shepherd, M., Goodman, N. & Watt, D.C. (1961). The application of hospital statistics in the evaluation of pharmacotherapy in a psychiatric population. *Comprehensive Psychiatry*, 2, 11–19.

Tooth, G. & Brooke, E. M. (1961). Mental hospital populations and their effect on future planning. *Lancet*, i, 710–13.

Watt, D. C. (1956). Reserpine and chlorpromazine in the treatment of chronic schizophrenics. *L'Encéphale*, 4, 601–2.

Watt, D. C. (1958). The effect of reserpine on the duration of manic attacks. *Journal of Neurology, Neurosurgery and Psychiatry*, 21, 297–300.

Watt, D. C. (1963*a*). The demand for psychiatric beds (letter). *Lancet*, i, 559.

Watt, D. C. (1963*b*). The demand for psychiatric beds (letter). *Lancet*, i, 997.

Watt, D. C. (1967*a*). Psychiatric beds (letter). *Lancet*, ii, 263–246.

Watt, D. C. (1967*b*). Psychiatric beds (letter). *Lancet*, ii, 512.

Watt, D. C., Allport, D. C. & Crookes, T.G. (1964). The effects of reserpine and chlorpromazine on stimulus-satiation and distractibility in human subjects. *Neuropsychopharmacology*, 3, ed. P. B. Bradley, F. Flügel & P. Hoch, pp. 93–9. In Proceedings of the 4th Meeting of the Collegium Internationale Neuropsychopharmacologicum. Amsterdam: Elsevier.

Watt, D. C. & Buglass, D. (1966). The effect of clinical and social factors on the discharge of chronic psychiatric patients. *Social Psychiatry*, 1, 57–63.

Watt, D. C., Crammer, J. L. & Elkes, A. (1972). Rate of metabolism and therapeutic response to desmethylimipramine. In *Societas Pharmacologica Hungarica V Conferentia Hungarica Pro Therapia et Investigatione in Pharmacologia*, pp. 125–31, Budapest, 1971.

Watt, D. C. & Crookes, T. G. (1961). The effect of reserpine on perceptual performance in human subjects. In *Neuropsychopharmacology*, 2, ed. E. Rothlin, pp. 410–13. In Proceedings of 2nd International Meeting of the Collegium Internationale Neuropsychopharmacologicum, Basle, 1960. Amsterdam: Elsevier.

Watt, D. C. Crookes, T. G. & McDonald, K. G. (1966). The reduction of reactive inhibition by reserpine in manic subjects. Proceedings of the 5th International Congress of Collegium Internationale Neuropsychopharmacologicum, p. 1069. Amsterdam: Elsevier.

Watt, D. C. & Shepherd, M. (1956). Chlorpromazine and Reserpine in chronic schizophrenia. A controlled clinical study. *Journal of Neurology, Neurosurgery and Psychiatry*, 19, 232–5.

Watt, D. C. & Shepherd, P. D. W. (1949). Curare-modified electric convulsion therapy in cases with physical disease. *British Medical Journal*, i, 752–63.

Weiskrantz, L. (1957). Reserpine and behavioural non-reactivity. In *Psychotropic Drugs*, ed. S. Garattini & V. Ghetti, pp. 67–72. Amsterdam: Elsevier.
Weiskrantz, L, & Wilson, W. A. (1955). The effects of reserpine on emotional behaviour of normal and brain-operated monkeys. *Annals of the New York Academy of Sciences,* 61, 36–55.
World Health Organisation (1978). *Mental Disorders; Glossary and Guide to their Publication in Accordance with the 9th Revision of the International Classification of Diseases.* Geneva: W.H.O.

Select bibliography

See also publications by D. C. Watt in References, pp. 200–1.

Watt, D. C. (1957). Suppression of the toxic effects of reserpine with phenidylate in chronic schizophrenia. *Report on the 2nd International Congress for Psychiatry, Zurich*, September 1957, 2, 394.
Watt, D. C., Crammer, J. L. & Elkes, A. (1968). The relation of side-effects to therapeutic response to desmethylimipramine. *Excerpta Medica International Congress Series, No. 180*, Proceedings of the VI International Congress of the Collegium Internationale Neuropsychopharmacologicum. Tarragona, April 1968. Amsterdam: Elsevier.
Watt, D. C. (1969). *Specific Treatment in Depression.* Oxford, London & Edinburgh: *Blackwell Scientific Publications*.
Watt, D. C., Brouckova, V., Bastecky J. & Velek, M. (1970). Drug addiction – a menace to youth in Great Britain. *Activitas Nervosa Superior*, 12-3, 284–7.
Watt, D. C. (1972). *OP Treatment of Schizophrenia with Long-acting Neuroleptics*. World Psychiatric Association, Symposium on Schizophrenia. Royal College of Physicians, London, 15 November 1972.
Watt, D. C., Crammer, J. L. & Elkes, A. (1972). Metabolism, anticholinergic effects and therapeutic outcome of desmethylimipramine. *Psychological Medicine*, 2, 397–405.
Watt, D. C. & Barraclough, B. (1972). Clinical Tutors in Psychiatry, Clinical Tutor's Sub-committee of the Royal Medico-Psychological Association. Reviewed in *Psychological Medicine*, 2, 200.
Watt, D. C. & Shepherd, M. (1974). Impact of long-term neuroleptics on the community: advantages and disadvantages. *Excerpta Medica International Congress Series No. 359, Neuropsychopharmacology*. Proceedings of the IX Congress of the Collegium Internationale Neuropsychopharmacologicum, Paris, 7–12 July 1974, ed. J. R. Boissier, H. Hippins & P. Pichot, pp. 379–82. Amsterdam: Excerpta Medica.
Watt, D. C. (1974). Depression – problems of treatment. *Modern Medicine*, 19, 111.
Watt, D. C. (1975). *Psychiatric Case Registers*. On Call, Feb. 18, p.6 Review of the Proceedings of the Conference on Psychiatric Case Registers, at the University of Aberdeen, 1974. HMSO.
Watt, D. C. (1975). Editorial: Time to evaluate long-acting neuroleptics? *Psychological Medicine*, 5, 222–6.

Watt, D. C. (1977). The relation of deviant symptoms and behaviour in a normal population to subsequent delinquency and maladjustment. *Psychological Medicine*, 7, 163–9.

Watt, D. C. (1977). Is an oral neuroleptic suitable for continuing drug treatment in schizophrenia? In Supplement 10, *Schizophrenia: Dopaminergic Mechanisms, Aetiology and Therapeutics: Some Questions Answered. Proceedings of the Royal Society of Medicine*, 70, 30–2.

Watt, D. C. & Shepherd, M. (1977). Long-term treatment with neuroleptics in psychiatry. In *Current Developments in Psychopharmacology, 4*, ed. W. B. Essmann & L. Valzelli, ch. VIII, pp. 217–47. New York: Spectrum Publications, Inc.

Watt, D. C. (1979). Are major drugs being prescribed for minor illnesses? *Mims Magazine*, 5–7, 15 June.

Watt, D. C. & Szulecka, T. K. (1979). The effect of sex, marriage and age at first admission on the hospitalisation of schizophrenics during 2 years following discharge. *Psychological Medicine*, 9, 529–40.

AUTHOR INDEX

SUBJECT INDEX

Subject Index

Subject Index

Subject index